Hi J...
"John" tells ME you are

FABULOUS After 50

God Bless
Shirley W Mitchell

2013

FABULOUS After 50

Shirley W. Mitchell

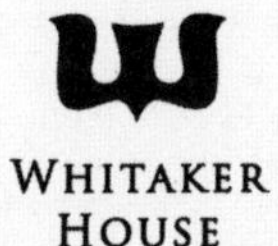

WHITAKER HOUSE

This information is not intended as a substitute for the personalized medical advice of your own physician. Women should regularly consult a physician in all matters relating to their health, particularly regarding any symptoms that may require diagnosis or medical attention.

FABULOUS AFTER 50

Shirley W. Mitchell
www.fabulousafter50.com

ISBN: 978-1-60374-737-0
eBook ISBN: 978-1-60374-738-7
Printed in the United States of America

Whitaker House
1030 Hunt Valley Circle
New Kensington, PA 15068
www.whitakerhouse.com

Library of Congress Cataloging-in-Publication Data

Mitchell, Shirley.
Fabulous after 50 / Shirley W. Mitchell.
pages cm
Originally published in Green Forest, AR by New Leaf Press, c2000.
Includes bibliographical references.
ISBN 978-1-60374-737-0—ISBN 978-1-60374-738-7 1. Middle-aged women—Religious life. 2. Christian women—Religious life. 3. Middle-aged persons—Religious life. I. Title. II. Title: Fabulous after fifty.
BV4579.5.M57 2013
248.8'5—dc23
2013015565

1 2 3 4 5 6 7 8 9 10 11 WH 19 18 17 16 15 14 13

DEDICATION

To Karen, David, Angela, and Jay–I'm proud to be your mom–and to Michelle, Monica, Melissa, Stephanie, Sarah, and Jackson–the greatest grandchildren in the universe.

–Shirley W. Mitchell

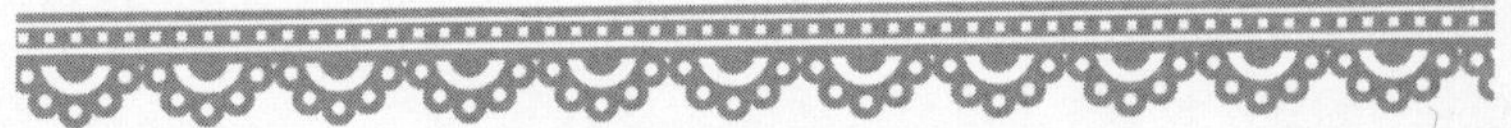

ACKNOWLEDGMENTS

I would like to express my appreciation to the following extremely special people who have helped me age sunny-side up and write this book to encourage others:

Willie Todd, my mother, for making me feel special, giving me her total love and attention, and implanting in me self-confidence and the ability to live to the max.

Karen Corcoran, my only daughter, for being a total woman of high spirits, drop-dead good looks, superintelligence, and true love.

David Mitchell, my oldest son, for having a pervasive sense of calm and wisdom. You are my rock.

Angela Mitchell, for filling our family with her exuberance for life.

Jay Mitchell, my youngest son, for being a man of integrity, having a warm heart, and lighting up my life.

Jack Mitchell, for sharing the great privilege of being parents and grandparents.

Michelle, Monica, Melissa, Stephanie, Sarah, and Jackson, for being the greatest grandchildren a grandmother could ever have.

Dr. James C. Upchurch, GYN, who caught the vision for this book in the beginning stages. Thanks, Jim, for adding expert information and much-needed encouragement.

Debra Goodwin, my sister, for adding excitement and knowledge to my life and this book.

Robert O., of Robert O. Studios, for his superb photography.

Dr. Ken Dychtwald, for giving me a new image of aging and a vision for *Fabulous After 50,* when I attended his Age Wave Institute in 1993 in New York City. Thanks, Dr. Dychtwald, for your great books *The Age Wave* and *Age Power.*

Dr. Walter M. Bortz II, for encouraging me to live an ageless life through his books, *We Live Too Short and Die Too Long* and *Dare to Be 100.* Dr. Bortz is responsible for my belief that I have the opportunity to age with good health, zeal, and power.

Gay N. Martin, author of *Alabama Off the Beaten Path, Louisiana Off the Beaten Path,* and *Alabama's Historic Restaurants and Their Recipes*; along with Alice Ducket, writer, columnist, and educator, for being my encouragers through our stimulating writers' critique group.

My extended family, Roy and Barbara Todd and Debra and Philip Goodwin, for loving and supporting me.

My super friends Carolyn Joseph, Linda Springfield, Pat Kennedy, Virginia Oliver, Jane Rubietta, Suzanne Block, and Elizabeth McLane, for being my soul mates.

O. E. Cruiser Small, my Agent-Producer, for his total dedication and love for this project.

—Shirley W. Mitchell

CONTENTS

The Ageless Woman's Pledge

The ageless woman
pledges,
regardless of the past:

to feel,
to laugh,
to grieve,
to forgive,
to grow,
to change,
to be willing to be wrong,
to touch,
to serve,
to love.

This woman leaves
a trail of grace
and a legacy of joy,
at any age!

–Jane Rubietta

For Shirley W. Mitchell,
my role model in victorious aging

PREFACE

TORCHBEARERS INTO THE FUTURE

Four weeks before the opening of the Olympic Games, a lighted torch—a stick of wood dipped in tallow or oil and set ablaze at the end to provide light that can be carried about—is brought by relay runners from the valley of Olympia, Greece, where the original Games were held, to the host country. Ships and planes transport the Olympic torch over the seas and mountains.

At the opening ceremony, the final runner carries the torch into the stadium, makes a dramatic lap around the track, followed by all of the other participating athletes, and then lights the Olympic flame. As the flame transfers from the runner's torch to the stationary torch, the Olympic Games officially begin.

Fabulous After 50, written in the crucible of life, aims to ignite aging women with a passion to shape and change the future because we dare to dream. The flame of the future is a new mental posture for women that enables them to feel younger while growing older and to get better while aging.

The objective of *Fabulous After 50* is to provide emotional, spiritual, and psychological wisdom, support, and guidance for women moving into the second half of life. This book addresses every woman's longing to impact the lives of others, to make every moment count, and to leave a legacy of love. Through this book and the attitude it fosters, I hope to defy society's bias that young is better. My desire is to give women mile markers for getting better, not just older, and to help all of us improve with age. To be enthusiastic about aging is almost an oxymoron; however, more and more mature women are becoming empowered to live their very best each day and are leading enjoyable, productive lives.

As expectations change for women, this book will propel them forward, clarify their calling, and give them more purposeful direction.

Fabulous After 50 covers a wide range of issues that concern women. This is a bookstore in a book, covering emotional and spiritual issues, as well as physical realities, such as proper diet, exercise, hormones, and menopause. Extensive research from secular and Christian sources gives balance to this book. At the end of each chapter is a section called "Questions for Immediate Application" to help women apply the practical principles from this book to their personal lives. This section also makes the book appropriate for discussions in the context of a small group or Bible study.

Chapter 9, "In the Jaws of Menopause," is an actual interview with James C. Upchurch, GYN., M.D., conducted as he guided me successfully through my own menopause. It will offer fresh hope as you approach this often-dreaded time.

My sister, Debra K. Goodwin, Registered Dietitian, guided me into healthy eating habits for a mature woman, and she will guide you, too, in chapter 7, "Debunking the Diet Mysteries: Eating Right."

After attending Dr. Ken Dychtwald's Age Wave Institute in New York, I caught his passion for making the latter years super years. The seed planted there in my fertile mind germinated into this book. Dr. Walter M. Bortz II, author of *We Live Too Long and Die Too Short* and *Dare to Be 100*, put an indelible groove into my brain to "use it or lose it."

I am delighted to invite you to run with the torch of ageless living into the future. I hope you will find life is truly *Fabulous After 50*.

CHAPTER 1

MAKE MIDLIFE PRIME TIME WITH A POSITIVE ATTITUDE TOWARD AGING

"As Boomers shed the skin of youth...they could be migrating into the most powerful years of their lives."[1]

—Dr. Ken Dychtwald, *Age Power*

"For as he thinketh in his heart, so is he."

—Proverbs 23:7 (KJV)

My best friend, Sarah, bounded up the steps of the jumbo jet, her agile body impressing me with its youthfulness. She appeared ageless. Sarah stopped at the top of the steps, turned, and smiled blithely. With a spirit of freedom, she waved and disappeared through the door of the plane.

Only I knew of the fierce struggle she'd encountered at midlife. Physical and emotional changes, including the darkness of depression, were now illuminated by energy, passion, and purpose. Opening the jaws of menopause and midlife had made her feel whole again, like a real woman. She even felt feminine. With the wisdom accrued from half a century of living, and with fewer family responsibilities, giving her more freedom to do the things she enjoyed, Sarah had begun experiencing the brightness and benefits of midlife.

> Probably the happiest period in life most frequently is in middle age, when the eager passions of youth are cooled, and the infirmities of age not yet begun; so we see that the shadows, which are at morning and evening so large, almost entirely disappear at mid-day.[2]

Sarah, in choosing to be fabulous after 50, defies the most common misconception of midlife.

• THE MISCONCEPTION ABOUT MIDLIFE •

In a society that values youth and beauty, people often think of midlife as the time when the quality of both life and the body begin to deteriorate. We focus on a sagging jaw line, age spots, or a body that is constantly moving closer to the ground. But life is more than what we see, and life can be better after 50! Growing older can be fabulous if we approach this mile marker relying on the wisdom we have gained. Centuries ago, Publilius Syrus said, "It takes a long time to bring excellence to maturity." Maturity and wisdom elevate us to a higher plateau in life for even greater contributions to our families, neighbors, societies, and communities, as well as to our local church.

These are the proving years—the years when we reap the benefits of living well and thoughtfully. As Jane O'Reilly put it,

> Fifty is a time of final options, but it is also a culmination, the prime of life, the beginning of seeing how it all turns out. Let there be less marveling at our wonderful preservation and more respect for the maturity of our mind and spirit. After all, the most important mission of a woman's life is not to hold on to her looks. Our mission is the same as a man's...to grow up. To ignore that goal is to exclude women from adult responsibility. Fifty

> is 50, and to deny that is to deny wisdom, experience and life itself.[3]

Perhaps, if you are approaching middle age, you are riding the waves of change that occur during this period, and feeling insecure. You may even be in the golden years, typically defined as age 65 and on. Despite changes in roles, careers, health, and relationships, we can always choose our outlook on aging and the many facets of growing older.

• POSITIVE AGING •

Dr. Ken Dychtwald has pioneered today's concept of aging. He is president and CEO of Age Wave, Inc., an education and communications firm that advises industry and government on the social, lifestyle, and business implications of an aging America. He said,

> I've spent the last 20 years studying aging and older people....When I got involved in the aging field it was primarily concerned with the sorrows and woes of aging. And while the concern among the professionals in my field was real and important, it seemed to me that by primarily focusing on the difficulties of aging—the terrible problems and enfeeblements that later years may bring—we were not hearing from the other voice, the voice of a more positive aging. There are people in this country growing old well—with vigor, with power, with style, with an interest in living fully and being part of the American marketplace.[4]

His term "Age Wave" refers to the huge demographic shift beginning in 1996, when the leading edge of the baby boomers—the 76 million people born between 1946 and 1964—turned 50 and merged with seniors to create an enormous senior society. Now, with millions of Americans over 50, positive aging is vital. In fact, there are more people over the age of 65 in the world today than at any other time in the history of the world put together.[5]

Einstein said, "Do not grow old, no matter how long you live. Never cease to stand like curious children before the Great Mystery into which we are born." Whatever your age, it's important to know that within every aging person lies hidden wealth.

• MINING FOR GOLD •

Like an unmined shaft, our depths gleam with nuggets of greatness. But having the potential for extraordinary achievements isn't enough; gold does the mine owner little good locked deep inside the earth's darkness. The nuggets must be mined, brought to the surface, taken through the fires of adversity, and polished to their peak of brilliance. This is no easy process. The refining process is difficult and painful, as Margaret Sharpe relates:

> For six thousand dollars worth of gold, it was most unremarkable looking stuff, like coarse black-speckled sand in a Ziplock sandwich bag. It glinted only dully in the brilliant sunshine, giving no hint of its potential to look anything like the glittering baubles we see in the windows of jewelry shops.
>
> After letting me feel the extraordinary weight of it, the prospector tossed the bag casually onto the dashboard of his pickup. It was his cut of the profits from a claim on Bonanza Creek which he was renting to another outfit.
>
> I thought of a few lines from Robert Service's poem "The Spell of the Yukon":

I wanted the gold, and I sought it;
I scrabbled and mucked like a slave.
Was it famine or scurvy—I fought it;
I hurled my youth into a grave.

I said, "So is this the stuff that men went mad trying to find?"

He gave a wry grin. "They still do. Everyone who comes here dreams of making it big."

We drove to the local assaying and concentrating company—a couple of trailers and a plywood and plastic shack just off the main road. There the gold was weighed and later would be refined. The young man in charge was about to melt down another lot. His furnace consisted of an old propane gas cylinder with the top sawn off, connected to a tank of compressed gas. There was a lengthy wait as the mixture of propane and oxygen was lit and the furnace came up to temperature, glowing a fiery orange-red.

He mixed the unrefined gold in a crucible with—of all things—borax, and placed it in the furnace. When he poured the molten gold into a bar mould, a thick black scum hardened on the surface. This he knocked off with a hammer once the bar was solid. I expected to see a gleaming bar of pure gold, but it was dull with black and grayish speckles. "There's still some iron in it," he said, "I'll have to do it again."

While this was going on, a far less dramatic method of gold separation continued inside the plywood shelter. Utterly ordinary-looking sand, the residue of bigger refining operations, was poured through a hopper onto a constantly vibrating table, where several minerals, including gold dust as fine as flour, were separated by specific gravity.

I couldn't imagine anything further removed from the activity of the massive bulldozers and sluicing machines we had seen operating out at Bonanza Creek itself, yet the goal was the same—to separate the gold from the worthless rock in which it is embedded, and to purify it.

There is nothing nice about the refining process. It is a dirty, messy job. The dross does not fall off but must be knocked off, piece by piece. Bulldozing ore produces tons of waste rock for each tiny ingot which is recovered. Even separating gold dust from sand requires a constant sweeping away of worthless minerals. The rewards for all that effort are certainly tangible for a successful prospector, who can hold six thousand dollars' worth of gold in the palm of his hand.

But God says that faith is more precious than gold which is perishable, even though tested by fire. Such faith is placed, not in the glittering brightness of gold or any other temporary thing, but in the eternal person and work of Jesus Christ, obtaining as the outcome of your faith the salvation of your souls...knowing that you were not redeemed with perishable things like silver or gold, but with the precious blood, as of a lamb unblemished and spotless, the blood of Christ. (See 1 Peter 1:7, 18–19.)

God often uses the idea of refining precious metals as a picture of what he does to get rid of the dross in our lives—whether it be our pride, our lust, our love of material things—whatever keeps us from acknowledging our need for His love and forgiveness. He considers the effort worthwhile, for the Bible tells us that Jesus, for the joy set before Him, endured the cross, despising the shame. (See Hebrews 12:2.)

If you have placed your faith and trust in Him, you are a gift of God to His glorious Son, the Creator and Sustainer of the universe. And He holds you in the palms of His hands, as infinitely more precious than gold.[6]

Unlike the so-called Gold Rush, where only an estimated thousand people actually struck gold, as we enter midlife we discover the vein of gold, the potential, running through every ageless person. We'll want to prospect! Digging and refining may look like revamping our vision, attaining a new understanding of our life purpose and gaining a revised outlook on the aging process.

In *Fabulous After 50*, we'll examine together the golden nuggets—the hidden wealth—of aging.

• REMOVING THE DROSS •

This wealth, unfortunately, is often hidden in the dross of a defeatist attitude. Just as gravity, sun, and time wrinkle the skin, so depression, worry, a broken spirit, and failure to dream can wrinkle the soul. Just because our eyesight is getting worse and our bodies are moving slowly south doesn't mean our spirits must drag lower and lower, as well.

At 50, we have unlimited potential to be fabulous, both of countenance and of spirit. We can make the most of the bodies and physical features we have—think of the value of a smile, regardless of wreaths of wrinkles!—while exercising great control over our spirit. Godly, healthy living, plus a positive attitude toward aging, can clear a path to fulfillment, happiness, health, and a rewarding state of satisfaction.

• THE KEY TO AGELESS LIVING •

Aging is inevitable. As we age, it is possible to sparkle like a jewel in the sun. With the proper mind-set, a positive attitude, a transcendent faith, and a practice of personal excellence, we'll become brighter. The marriage of experience and mature faith gives us the opportunity to enjoy a rich older life. Trusting God is the key to ageless living. In times of insecurity and fear, which seem to increase with age, I know I must trust God.

Don't allow the "old lady syndrome" to make you a shadow of the woman you are or could be. Some of our best and brightest women, though past the half-century mark in years, are climbing the ladder of success in the world—and the Stairmaster at the gym. This is the time to be bold, self-assured, empowered, and socially and politically aware. Viewing this time in our lives as a renewal is one way.

Renewal

Life is a series of renewals. Each morning opens the door on a fresh, just-born day. I take the gift of each sunrise as a new beginning, a time for God to renew me. Birthdays, too, can be renewals, offering the chance to start fresh with a clean slate, to revamp, to choose new areas of growth and exploration. Remember a "sweet 16"? To the teenager receiving her first driver's license, the world is bright and new and made just for her. Graduation, a further milestone along the lifeline, opens door after door to new starts: career, marriage, and family.

This is why Gail Sheehy calls midlife a "second adulthood." Middle age is another time of renewal in life, a season that may lead us to different activities, higher goals, and deeper relationships. And this is just the beginning!

Adventure

Turning a midlife crisis into a quest can be a special journey of new beginnings. Aging can be a voyage of discovery! After all, it wasn't until Christopher Columbus was in his early 40s that he made his first voyage to America. He made his voyage for God... for gold. When we adopt Christopher Columbus' adventurous spirit, our midlife years can have the Midas touch.

Dreaming is central to approaching midlife as an adventure. To begin this adventure, we must go to the nucleus of our hearts and spirits to let the real person shine through. By learning to listen to our heart's desires and allowing our Creator to be our compass, each of us will find our own guideposts of fulfillment as we follow our dreams. God has a special plan for each life, and He plants within us a dream to pursue it. Even after 50 years of life, we can begin to dream again.

A Race

In the Bible, the apostle Paul compares life to a race, in which we are all striving to obtain an incorruptible crown:

> *In a race, everyone runs but only one person gets first prize. So run your race to win. To win the contest you must deny yourselves many things that would keep you from doing your best. An athlete goes to all this trouble just to win a blue ribbon or a silver cup, but we do it for a heavenly reward that never disappears. So fight to win. I'm not just shadow-boxing or playing around. Like an athlete I punish my body, treating it roughly, training it to do what it should, not what it wants to. Otherwise, I fear that after enlisting others for the race, I myself might be declared unfit and ordered to stand aside.*
>
> (1 Corinthians 9:24–27 TLB)

While we're for the gold, however, the course in the aging race may well change! Previous generations followed what is called a linear lifestyle—moving through youth, getting an education, working at a single career until 65, and then rocking away in retirement while waiting for death. Recently, this linear lifestyle has fallen out of fashion. Retirement is a new concept, which may have contributed to the devaluing of aging people. B.F. Skinner made this point, saying,

> For many people, old age begins with retirement.... Retirement is a modern idea. Until recently, as people grew older they simply did less and less of what they had always done, or turned to work that was easier. In 1870, in America, only one-quarter of the men over sixty-five were not working. A hundred years later, this figure was three-quarters. American women are "retiring" sooner, too. When families were larger, parents might be in their sixties before the last child left home. Today they may be no more than forty-five. When old age starts that soon, it lasts a long time.[7]

On the contrary, the cyclic lifestyle depicts a more helpful, healthful circular path, where one is free to begin again. And again. We may launch a new career or enter into a new personal relationship, maybe forging a whole new life in a new place during middle age. This cyclic lifestyle, and a new paradigm—that older is better—are sending many older women out to search for a new identity of power, style, and vigor.

Alice exemplifies this cyclic lifestyle. Her laser listening enabled her to hear the whisper of a dream in her heart. Though enjoying notable success in the educational field, she anticipates retirement with enthusiasm. Her passions for reading, writing, and traveling are coming together in a new dream career. She has mapped out plans for this adventure by combining her interests and becoming a travel writer. Her mind is exploding with ideas and possibilities for the future. Her dreams have not turned gray or become wrinkled but rather are fresh, new, and vibrant.

Along with an enticing career change, this middle-aged lady is experiencing the great adventure of being a grandmother. For her, the autumn of life offers the prospect of being exciting, different, and even better than the first half.

A New Season

My home state of Alabama puts on a dazzling show during the fall season. God takes His brush and paints the leaves vibrant hues of scarlet, deep purple, sunshine yellow, and glowing orange. The landscape is as beautiful as a postcard. Just as the autumn of the year splashes bright colors everywhere, so does the autumn of life. Step out from the drab dryness of late summer to the color, panache, and wonder of this extraordinary life season!

Joseph Antonini, former chairman and CEO of K-Mart Corporation, said, "Life stage is more important than age!"

Carolyn Miller believes this to be true. The 1996 national president of the Southern Baptist Women's Missionary Union agrees that life's stage—the quality of life and contributions made—is much more important than years lived.

Carolyn and I grew up together. We attended church each Sunday, giggling and whispering in the pews, then headed to her home. I would eat lunch with her family, and then we'd sprawl on the floor in front of the roaring fireplace and play Monopoly. Her spacious home was warm with love. In the evening, we always returned to church for the young people's group.

Four decades later, we reunited for lunch. The years that had passed vanished like snow under the intense heat of sunshine as Carolyn and I caught up on the intervening time. She shared about her travels and her work helping women around the nation.

"What do you think is the secret of women being 'fabulous after 50'?" I asked her.

"Love God, love yourself, love people." She smiled. "I like people who are so inwardly fabulous that I don't see their outside appearance. Likewise, I have met people who are fabulous-looking but are shallow on the inside. Age and external beauty are irrelevant to the fabulous after-50 woman.

"Fabulous women are good listeners and givers. They enjoy a balanced life. Fabulous 50-plus women will be imitators of Christ and also His ambassadors."

Looking at this fabulous woman across the table, I knew she lived out her own philosophy. Her travels throughout the world, making speeches and attending countless committee meetings and functions, had forced her to live with integrity while continuing her career as a wife, mother, grandmother, and homemaker. Her ageless appeal broadened her meaningful contribution to the 1.7 million-member women's group. She impressed me as a gracious lady whose real strength comes from the substance of her soul.

Leaving the restaurant that day, I realized Carolyn embraced life with exuberance. Undoubtedly she will relish it and live it to the fullest, giving no thought to age by numbers. Life is a stage, not an age. Putting God in the center of the stage to direct life at middle age—and at every age—is a win-win casting decision.

Carolyn's brightness reminds me that age doesn't dull our luster, because the shine comes from within, from the "*hidden person of the heart*" (1 Peter 3:4).

To keep your life from losing its luster in middle age, try to maintain a positive attitude based on the following proclamations:

1. I will stay young at heart. I will keep growing and going.
2. On my journey beyond youth, I will stay young at heart by living the moment, laughing, and embracing a positive attitude.
3. My personal relationship with Jesus Christ will empower me to experience the beauty of being an ageless person.
4. Knowing God through a daily time of quiet intimacy propels my life into universal and eternal living. It gives me wings to fly through my maturing life and reason to live well.
5. I will choose to live fully after 50, dreaming new dreams and investing my energies to the lives of others.
6. Investing in relationships for eternity gives life depth, breadth, and a reason for living well.
7. Excellent nutrition energizes me to live agelessly.
8. With proper exercise, I can rekindle my fire for life.
9. I will open the jaws of menopause with help from my doctor, great habits, and a great attitude.
10. To be 50ish, female, and fabulous, I will make the most of my best.
11. I will dance with anticipation every day of my life as I move toward eternity and my final home.

Fabulous After 50 is your personal invitation to a lifelong, and long-life, celebration. Congratulations! You are a woman of strength! You have survived disease and accidents. Taking God's free gift of time and adding increased strength, faith, and new dreams will give renewed life to our remaining years.

How old would you be if you didn't know how many years you had already lived? Your answer will help determine the quality of life to the end of your days. Youth has far more to do with mind and spirit than years lived. As Max Lucado said, "Your goal is not to live long; it's to live."

I suggest that we set our minds at "young" and keep going. The ancient King Solomon reminds us that what you think is what you are. (See Proverbs 23:7.) Far too many women over 50 feel old, useless, and depleted. A small percent grab life and go with it. I want us as women to feel precious, empowered, and encouraged as we embrace our middle years.

Let's walk arm in arm into the future filled with hope. Every day of midlife will offer abundant adventure and excitement if we maintain the right perspective.

• QUESTIONS FOR IMMEDIATE APPLICATION •

1 List five things you choose to do in your own personal life that will make your midlife prime time.
2. Write down (a) a higher goal, (b) a new activity, and (c) a deeper relationship that will renew your "second adulthood."
3. What do you think is the secret of being fabulous after 50?

• TEN WAYS TO CHEAT AGING •

1. *Believe*—in God; faith keeps you sipping from the Fountain of Youth. Women who have faith and attend worship service regularly live longer and better.
2. *Exercise*—Use it or lose it! Exercise your body, soul, spirit, and mind.
3. *Attitude*—We are what we think. Some of us are growing younger, but most of us are growing older. If we work with energy and zeal, expecting life to be rich, full, and adventurous, that expectation will be a self-fulfilling prophecy.

4 *Maintain Proper Diet*—A daily balanced diet from the "Food Guide Pyramid" (you can find it on your bread wrapper!). Take one multivitamin/multi-mineral dietary supplement daily.

5. *Laugh*—Women who laugh, last! Laughter is a stress buster that lifts both our spirits and our faces. It juices the chemical endorphins in the brain, which make us feel euphoric.

6. *Keep Moving*—Get up and go! If you dread growing older because you fear physical deterioration and memory loss, your fears will likely be realized. However, if you use this time to keep moving and growing, you prescribe for yourself years of excitement and adventure.

7. *Look Good*—When you look your best, you feel your best, and you receive more positive response from the people with whom you interact.

8. *Live in the Now*—Live your best now. Each new day is a new chance at life. Yesterday is a cancelled check. Tomorrow is a promissory note. Today is a check. Have fun spending it.

9. *Rekindle*—Make your aging life burn with energy. It takes only a spark to get a fire going.

10. *Give*—You can't out-give God or people.

• THE ABC'S OF AGING GRACEFULLY •

A—Attitude

B—Beauty goes beyond looks

C—Church

D—Diet

E—Exercise

F—Fiber! Fearless! Forgiveness!

G–Gravity isn't for the heart

H–Help others

I–Ideas and ideals

J–Joy

K–Kindness

L–Learn constantly; listen; look

M–Motivation; mind over matter

N–Notice

O–Out with osteoporosis

P–Prevention

Q–Quit bad habits

R–Read

S–Stress reduction; soul care

T–Treasure others

U–Understanding

V–Volunteer; values

W–Walk; work; wonder; wisdom

X–(These are always contrived) How about x-perience? x-citement?

Y–Youthful heart

Z–Zeal, zero gravity

AGING SUCCESSFULLY: ATTITUDE #1

I will set my mind at "young" and keep going and growing.

CHAPTER 2

FIGHTING MIDLIFE FEARS

"Who well lives, long lives; for this age of ours should not be numbered by years, days, and hours."

—Guillaume de Salluste,
Divine Weeks and Works, Book 2

William James, the 18th-century philosopher, said, "It is attitude at the beginning of a difficult undertaking which, more than anything else, will determine its successful outcome."

Whatever our place in the middle-age race, it is never too late to face our fears about aging in order to embrace a positive attitude and make the most of every day.

Aging is no longer considered a time in life to fight against or to fear. Aging is a natural part of the growth process, one that is lengthening and improving with medical and social advances. In addition, fear is not of God. He gives us a spirit of power, love, and sound mind. (See 2 Timothy 1:7.) When we are full of love, power, and a sound mind, there is no room for fear.

Rev. Peter Lord, speaking at a conference at Park Avenue Baptist Church in Titusville, Florida, stated, "Fear is the darkroom where negatives are developed."

As we become surfers on the "age wave," the fears of middle age will dissolve. Some of these fears and questions include:

1. Can life be good during and after middle age?
2. Can I be young in my mind?
3. Physically, mentally, socially, spiritually–will I have zeal for life?
4. Will I survive the "jaws of menopause"?
5. Can I have an exciting sex life after menopause?
6. Will exercise keep me younger in body, as the "golden egg" of aging?
7. Will I be able to keep my family ties strong?
8. Can I be loving–and loved–as I age and my body changes?
9. What meaningful contributions will I make in this "second adulthood"?
10. Is it possible to know God and face death with faith?
11. Is there a heaven?

• FIGHT FEAR WITH LIVING WATER •

These fears need not submerge us. When age bumps into our youth, threatening to drown us in fear, we can be empowered by a mental agenda that affirms we will be forever young. What we think, we bring about.

Why not search for the "fountain of youth"? Back through the pages of time, the placebo on those searching for this elusive fountain has caused a positive mind-set. Believing they found the secret to eternal youth, these adventurers lived young! This positive attitude, combined with a healthy lifestyle, goes a long way toward enabling us to feel and act young.

The sourcebook for life, the Bible, declares the fountain of youth to be spiritual, not physical. Our attitude has to do with our ways of thinking and feeling; our spirituality is the way we interact with God. Jesus Christ unlocks the secret of youth when He invites us to drink of the fountain of living water. He says, "*If anyone thirsts, let him come to Me and drink. He who believes in Me, as the Scripture has said, out of his heart will flow rivers of living water*" (John 7:37–38 NKJV).

• FIGHT FEAR WITH FOCUS •

One woman who unlocked the door to eternal youthfulness through a positive attitude and faith is Helen Keller. Being both blind and deaf, she had a legitimate excuse to do nothing with her life but complain and grow old. Yet she became an international symbol of strength, achievement, and encouragement. Despite her limitations, Helen Keller did not allow fear to incapacitate her. She urges us:

> Join the great company of those who make the barren places of life fruitful with kindness. Carry a vision of heaven in your hearts, and you shall make your name, your college, the world, correspond to that vision. Your success and happiness live in you. External conditions are the accidents of life, its outer wrappings. The great, enduring realities are love and service. Joy is the holy fire that keeps our purpose warm and our intelligence aglow. Resolve to keep happy, and your joy and you shall form an invincible host against difficulty.[1]

When our life focus moves from a self-centered preoccupation with our bodies and futures to an external focus that seeks to serve others, the opportunities are overwhelming. By embracing the twin purposes of joy and service, fear of aging is cast out, replaced with an ability to live wholly in the present.

• FIGHT FEAR BY LIVING IN THE MOMENT •

Father Time and Mother Nature do not sentence us to old age. Living old is a choice; and so is living young. The attitude that views each new day as a special gift will keep us sipping from the fountain of youth. Baby boomers are part of the "carpe diem" generation—they seize the day.

Every morning, we are handed a package of 1,440 new, unused minutes to be spent in the manner we choose. At the end of the day, those minutes are gone forever. We cannot bank them, save them, or carry them over to the next day.

"Each day is a new life," sang the gorgeous, radiant Kim Wimmer, crowned Miss Alabama in 1993. The opportunities of today will never be repeated. So, walk through every door with enthusiasm. A great way to start the day at the first awareness after a good night's sleep is to resolve, "*This is the day the Lord has made; we will rejoice and be glad in it*" (Psalm 118:24 NKJV).

In His infinite wisdom, the Creator gives us only one moment at a time. That's all we can handle! In an hourglass, one single grain of sand may slip through the narrow connecting tube of the glass at a time. As moments turn into days, the sands of time create, like sand in an oyster, the perfect chance to make each day into a pearl. At the end of our lives, if we have lived them fully, what a glowing strand of pearls we'll have! "Successful living, and happy aging, require that [we] live in the present and for the future rather than dwell on losses."[2]

• FIGHT FEAR WITH LEVITY •

The ageless woman gives God center stage. With God in the middle of our lives, we have the security to poke fun at aging, as did Dr. Penne Laubenthal in her poem "Mid-Life Crisis."

"MID-LIFE CRISIS"

Everyone I know is thirty-five.
Donna, in my writing class, is thirty-five.
Melissa, the artist, is thirty-five.
Only I am no longer thirty-five.

Last night when I was sleeping
someone slipped in and
scribbled lines all over my face,
stuck bags under my eyes,
packed cellulite on my thighs.

This morning my mother's hand reached
to get my toothbrush.
An unfamiliar face stared back at me
from the vanity,
someone else's stomach protruded
from beneath my belt.

The kudzu of middle-age has overtaken me.
Cholesterol clogs my arteries
like milfoil on the Tennessee River.
Yesterday I was thirty-five.
Today I am forty-five.

I had intended to age elegantly—
grow lean like Louise Nevelson,
craggy like O'Keefe,
not squat like Gertrude Stein.

Tomorrow I am going to buy a new mirror,
have my hair dyed,
phone about a facelift.

Meanwhile, I am going to claim
that my children belong to my husband
by a former marriage
and I am going to lie—
I am going to say
"I am only thirty-five."[3]

Living, dying, coping with change—these are the challenges of human existence, all of them very serious subjects indeed. But, in the bibliotherapy class Dr. Laubenthal teaches at Athens State College in Athens, Alabama, her students also experience the healing power of honest laughter and learn firsthand the value of humor in restoring balance and perspective to their lives. They laugh at stories, at each other, and at themselves.

Dr. Laubenthal led her class in a discussion of the book *Mirror Mirror: The Terror of Not Being Young* by Elissa Melamed. In the course of their discussion, Dr. Laubenthal made this candid admission:

> The blatant truth is that it is swimsuit season, and I am forced to face what I have so deftly hidden all winter long. Furthermore, I am approaching my forty-fifth birthday and unlike Jack Benny, I cannot go to my grave claiming to be thirty-nine.

It was after reading *Mirror Mirror* that Dr. Laubenthal wrote her poem "Mid-Life Crisis." When she shared it with her class, they all enjoyed a hearty laugh at one of our deepest fears: aging.

The professor said to me, "I don't pretend this therapeutic process made me feel any younger, but I do declare it made me feel better about being older!"

• FIGHT FEAR WITH LAUGHTER •

If you laugh, you last! A positive, youthful mind-set helps us lighten up and also lightens the load we haul around with us. Spontaneous humor invading our living gives life spice. Laughter is a stress buster, lifting both the spirits and the face. Laughter juices the chemical endorphins in the brain that make us feel euphoric.

In the movie *Patch Adams*, based on a true story, Robin Williams plays medical student Hunter "Patch" Adams, who fights against the traditional strictures of medicine with humor and patient empathy. Facing a supervisor who is angry about Adams's break with traditional medicine, Adams spouts that, according to the *American Journal of Medicine*,

> Laughter increases the secretion of endorphins, which in turn increases oxygenation of the blood, relaxes the arteries, speeds up the heart, decreases blood pressure, which has a positive effect on all cardiovascular and respiratory ailments as well as overall increasing the immune system response.

Though his supervisor was not impressed, his patients were, and Patch Adams's work led to the founding of a free hospital called The Geshundeit Institute, with a waiting list of thousands of physicians ready to provide free medical care to patients. Laughter has healing properties, proving the truth of wise old King Solomon's words: "*A cheerful merry heart does good, like medicine*" (Proverbs 17:22 NKJV).

Writes Frances Weaver, in *The Girls with the Grandmother Faces*, "The never-fail rule for feeling better about being older is maintaining a sense of humor."[4]

Laughter also gives us an ageless quality that knows no boundaries or limitations. Once again, we see the close connection between attitude and age. Richard Armour says, "I hope I have a young outlook. Since I have an old everything else, this is my one chance of having a bit of youth as a part of me."[5]

Age is just a number, and mine is not listed! Laughter keeps me young—I think young; I feel young. The intoxicating joy of growing old with Jesus Christ makes laughter come easily and lavishes a youthful dew over the 50-something woman. The fountain of aging overflows with savvy, well-educated, fulfilled women who can laugh at the days to come.

Glenn Van Ekeren relates the following story:

> One Sunday afternoon, a cranky grandfather was visiting his family. As he lay down to take a nap, his grandson decided to have a little fun by putting Limburger cheese on Grandfather's mustache. Soon, Grandpa awoke with a snort and charged out of the bedroom, saying, "This room stinks." Throughout the house he went, finding every room smelling the same. Desperately he made his way outside only to find that "the whole world stinks!"
>
> So it is when we fill our minds with negativism. Everything we experience and everybody we encounter will carry the scent we hold in our mind.[6]

As we march into the future, an increasing number of health professionals believe that living in the moment, laughing, and maintaining a positive attitude are vital habits of continuing good health.

"GROW OLDER WITHOUT GETTING OLD"

by Shirley W. Mitchell

The "age wave" is here,
that no one will deny.

The older crowd is growing,
it's our time to fly.

Exercise is the golden egg
that will reverse this aging.
We walk, we jog, we Jazzercise
to keep our energy raging.

With proper diet and attitude
we golden oldies believe
we retard the ravages
of age, gravity, and disease.

Jumping into the sea of aging
with wild anticipation,
exhilaration, excitement, and adventure
will be our reputation.

What's our secret
for growing older without getting old?
Positive thinking and enthusiasm
is the oldest secret ever told.

Jesus is the answer
as we walk this earthly road.
We're only getting better,
we're not getting old.

• QUESTIONS FOR IMMEDIATE APPLICATION •

1. How do you plan to fight your own midlife fears?
2. Second Timothy 1:7 tells us that God does not give us the spirit of fear. God gives us the spirit of _________, _________, and _________. How would you describe your spirit as you face midlife?

3. List three ways you will put more fun and laughter into your life.

• TOP TEN AUTOMATIC AGERS •

1. Fear of change
2. Worry
3. Negative thinking
4. A blaming spirit
5. Inability to be wrong
6. Narrow-mindedness
7. Forgetting to laugh
8. Failing to grieve
9. Poor self-care
10. Unforgiveness and bitterness

AGING SUCCESSFULLY: ATTITUDE #2

I will stay young at heart by living in the moment, laughing, and embracing a positive attitude.

CHAPTER 3

THE AGELESS WOMAN: LIVING VICTORIOUSLY IS POSSIBLE BY EMBRACING OUR SPIRITUALITY

"The light of Jesus shining through
an aging woman will make her sparkle.
Her life will shine forth the many facets of Jesus just as
a cut gem reflects beautiful color in all directions."[1]

–Shirley W. Mitchell,
Spiritual Sparks for Busy Women

"Charm can be deceptive and beauty doesn't last, but a woman who fears and reverences God shall be greatly praised."

–Proverbs 31:30 (TLB)

As I rode my bike down the rocky path to the barn, my long brown hair streamed in the wind while my fertilizer-bag dress flapped against my bony knees. I was 15 years old, the child of tenant cotton farmers; but, in my mind, I was rich. The night before, in the silence of my heart and the stillness of my bedroom, my life had changed for eternity. Though I had stitched my dress from a colorful, printed bag I'd retrieved from the field, my heart was wrapped in the robes of royalty.

• FERTILE SOIL •

We lived on a cotton farm in a square white house, with four equal rooms, built by my dad in the middle of the potato patch. We attended a small country church, and that week had been set aside for "Revival Services." Each year, the members of Mt. Vernon Church experienced a spiritual revival while learning the importance of being born into the family of God.

That hot August night, as I lay in my small, stuffy bedroom, the minister's words burned through my mind like the lights on my daddy's pickup truck. He had proclaimed from the pulpit, "'*For God so loved the world, that he gave his only begotten Son, that whosoever believeth in him should not perish, but have everlasting life*' (John 3:16 KJV)."

I had probably heard those words weekly for my entire childhood, but that night, they singed my soul, gripping me with an urgency to set things right. I remembered another Scripture from the pastor's message: "'*Come now, and let us reason together, saith the LORD: though your sins be as scarlet, they shall be as white as snow; though they be red like crimson, they shall be as wool*' (Isaiah 1:18 KJV)."

As I tossed and turned on my bed, the dreams and discontents of a teenager gave way to an even deeper urging to secure my soul for eternity with Christ. Drenched in the humid night air, I envisioned the white snow in Scripture and longed for that one-on-one relationship with Jesus, God's Son. All the loneliness, the pain, the poverty, and the hard work receded into the darkness as the light of God poured over me, and I said "Yes!" to Jesus.

The relief was instant. I knew that if I died before morning, I would go directly to heaven to be with Jesus and live forever. The minister had assured me that the blood of Jesus would wash me as white as snow, and I fell asleep, deeply loved and deeply loving God for the first time.

Now, 40 years later, this reality is still printed indelibly on my mind. I live with the luxury of being a member of the royal family of God.

• AGELESS LIVING •

Our lives have been rocked in the past years with the untimely deaths of prominent members of various royal families, from Princess Grace (Monaco) to the much-loved Princess Diana (Wales). Even our own American "royals" are not exempt from death—Jackie Kennedy Onassis died from cancer, and her son John was killed in a plane crash. As much as we have mourned their passing, we know that the secret to royal living does not come from our earthly parents or marrying into the right family.

The secret to being fabulous after 50 comes with being "born again" into the royal family of God, as a believer and as a child of the King. We can jump deeper into life with great anticipation, even if we are 50 years young, by nurturing an intimate relationship with God's Son, Jesus Christ.

This is truly ageless living. One must have the Spirit of God living inside, know God, and allow the Holy Spirit to guide, teach, and comfort. Knowing God is crucial to living successful lives.

Peggy Noonan, author of *Life, Liberty and the Pursuit of Happiness*, speaks for the baby boomer of the 21st century. As a speechwriter for former U.S. President Ronald Reagan, she went back to her Bible. In her book, she gives optimistic advice: "'...give your love and know your God and do your work. And be good to your troupe,' all those people who give your life meaning."[2]

Peggy Noonan has cut to the core of the baby boomer's search for truly successful aging. We get to know God through reading His living Word, the Holy Bible; praying (talking with and listening to God); and spending time with Him (practicing personal meditation).

We are cruel to ourselves if we try to live in this wild, mean world without knowing God the Father, God the Son, and God the Holy Spirit. People will disappoint and hurt us, but God, who created the earth, will not. He made you and me for His pleasure. "*Thou art worthy, O Lord, to receive glory and honour and power: for thou hast created all things, and for thy pleasure they are and were created*" (Revelation 4:11 KJV). We lose out when we don't take advantage of knowing the very Creator of the entire universe.

And when we disregard hearing God's Word, the Bible, we stumble and blunder around with no sense of direction. Without God, you and I will waste our lives, and lose our souls in the process.

What would you lose if you said yes to Jesus?

Nothing!

What would you gain?

Abundant, eternal life!

If you desire to be "fabulous after 50 and beyond" by becoming a born-again believer, pray this prayer in your heart:

> Jesus, I say "Yes" to You. I desire to be a member of the royal family of God. I turn from my sin to follow You. Cover my sins with the blood of Jesus and forgive me. Amen.

When we turn to God, we can count on the good news: "*If we confess our sins, He is faithful and righteous to forgive us our sins and to cleanse us from all unrighteousness*" (1 John 1:9).

• STAGES OF THE AGELESS CHRISTIAN LIFE •

Watching the beautiful, multicolored monarch butterfly flit from flower to flower, my spirit lightened. The soundless and unhurried movements of God's gorgeous creature gave the garden a sense of relaxation and timelessness. The dappled sunlight danced on the fragile wings, inspiring me.

My thoughts were caught up in the metamorphosis of this beautiful creature, from a tightly wrapped cocoon to a large, swollen body with tiny, shriveled wings, and finally to an exquisite, mature butterfly.

The Christian life with the life has many parallels to the life of a butterfly. In the "cocoon stage," we are born again, and Christ wraps us in His blanket of love. Then, we become hungry for God's voice, so we begin to study the Bible and communicate with Him through prayer, growing spiritually as a result. Like the butterfly in its swollen body/shriveled wings stage, through the struggle and pain of growth, in God's perfection and timing, we become mature Christians–beautiful like a monarch butterfly.

How does a mature Christian, like a butterfly, shed multicolored beams of God's love to her world? How does she let the beauty of God rest upon her?

I have found only one way–to do as the apostle James stated: "*Come near to God and he will come near to you*" (James 4:8 NIV). The delightful promise inherent in this Scripture is this: God obligates Himself to draw near to us in response. Because He has called us "royalty," we are drawn into His family.

> *But you are a chosen race, a royal priesthood,...a people for God's own possession, that you may proclaim the excellencies of Him who has called you out of darkness into His marvelous light.* (1 Peter 2:9)

• ROYALTY •

Being a member of a royal family is the fantasy of many teenagers. However, being a member of the universal "family of God" is mind-boggling!

Paul E. Billheimer, in his book *Destined for the Throne*, said, "Through the new birth a redeemed human being becomes a bona fide member of the original cosmic family, 'next of kin' to the Trinity."[3]

We are a lonely, disconnected society. Our hurry-worry pace creates isolation and loneliness. This "alone" feeling activates an urgent desire to link hands around the universe with others, being connected by God. As members of the universal "family of God," our numbers grow exponentially! Read some of Paul's words on the subject:

> *Those who are led by the Spirit of God are sons of God. For you did not receive a spirit that makes you a slave again to fear, but you received the Spirit of sonship. And by him we cry, "Abba, Father." The Spirit himself testifies with our spirit that we are God's children. Now if we are children, then we are heirs–heirs of God and co-heirs with Christ, if indeed we share in his sufferings in order that we may also share in his glory.*
>
> (Romans 8:14–17 NIV)

Times of perceived aloneness can become opportunities for the family of God to surround us. This has proven true for me countless times.

• THE RED ROSE •

Through blurred vision, the gorgeous, velvet red rose came gradually into focus. I had been sick with the flu, miserable and isolated for a week. Opening my eyes, I knew my sister, 15 years my junior, had slipped into my room while I was sleeping and left the long-stemmed beauty. The fact that she cared enough about me to visit my sickroom while I slept, leaving my favorite flower in a delicate vase, cheered my soul.

She is my sister, both biologically and in Christ, and she lights up my life. Her loving gift reminded me that I was not alone, and that "*whoever does the will of my Father in heaven is my brother and sister and mother*" (Matthew 12:50 NIV). The reminder that I was a "child of the King" who belonged to the universal "royal family" of God gave me eternal hope and raised my spirits, in spite of my illness.

The royal family of God may connect us around the world, but it also connects us right where we live.

• LOCAL CONNECTIONS •

As a member of this royal family, it is important to find a local church where you can worship God with other believers. The camaraderie of being a member of a local church dissolves loneliness. Your spiritual "siblings" will worship with you, rejoice with you, celebrate life with you, and be your burden bearers when times get tough!

Years ago, when I had a major surgery, the people around my hospital bed supporting me with love and prayer were my family, my pastor, the choir director from my church, and my sisters in Christ.

When times get tough, the royal family of God surrounds us with support. This is the way God makes His love real to us and meets our very real needs.

A young woman had just started attending a local church when her doctors ordered total bed rest for her problem pregnancy. The church learned about her dilemma and organized a group of people to help clean the house, care for her children, provide a meal every day, and run errands for the family. This young woman is now a member of the royal family of God. Why? Because her church congregation loved her into their family!

By accepting Christ's gift of salvation, we all have the right to live the robust, rich life of a child of the King! And as the King's children, we can face the future with courage and hope, because God has a pet name for us.

• PECULIAR TREASURES •

Thousands of years ago, God said to Moses, "*Now therefore, if ye will obey my voice indeed, and keep my covenant, then ye shall be a peculiar treasure unto me above all people: for all the earth is mine*" (Exodus 19:5 KJV). He speaks these same words to us, His children, today.

In studying the word *peculiar*, I learned it means personal, special, exceptional, particular, private, characteristic, exclusive, specific, unusual, uncommon, and rare.

Wow! God's children who hear His voice and keep His covenant are indeed important to Him! How precious it is to be a peculiar treasure to God!

Jesus lights a candle in the darkness of aging with bright optimism and hope for His peculiar treasures. "*You have turned on my light! The Lord my God has made my darkness turn to light*" (Psalm 18:28 TLB).

Though we have lived 50 years and made many mistakes, God still loves us. He has given us the free gifts of salvation and resurrection, and has promised us a place with Him in the heavenly realms. This amazing truth keeps me young and yearning for eternity!

• COLLECTIBLE JEWELS •

Beauty cuts into aging like light into shadow, making us like rare collectible jewels. Though beauty often moves inside older women, we can radiate the sparkling beauty of Jesus Christ. The beauty of being God's ageless woman is being beautiful inside and out through the positive power of Jesus Christ.

Listening to the radio one day, I heard a song that included this line: "I'm just an old chunk of coal, but I am going to be a diamond someday." The words reminded me that coal becomes diamonds only through intense pressure. Those lumps become sparkling and priceless through the hands of a master chiseler. My hope continues to be that someday God will make a diamond out of me.

God's Word tells us that He is "making up His jewels."

> *Then they that feared the LORD spake often one to another: and the LORD hearkened, and heard it, and a book of remembrance was written before him for them that feared the LORD, and that thought upon his name. And they shall be mine, saith the LORD of hosts, in that day when I make up my jewels; and I will spare them, as a man spareth his own son that serveth him.* (Malachi 3:16–17 KJV)

As we surrender our lives to Jesus, we become exquisite jewels. God's splendor shall sparkle from our lives, and we will be a light to others. The truly ageless woman's life will shine forth the many facets of Jesus, just as a cut gem reflects beautiful color in all directions. Age can grind us or shine us. Refuse to let the fear of aging dull your luster!

• A SHINING LIFE •

June Fricks radiates that sparkle. When the former sales director for the State Lodge in Lake Guntersville, Alabama, enters a room, her joy brightens the atmosphere. Like Jesus, she is "*clad with zeal as a cloak*" (Isaiah 59:17 KJV). Enthusiasm is the wellspring of her life, as evidenced through her ability to love and accept even the most difficult of people and work to make each event she booked a memorable one for all involved.

Being on the advisory board of the Congressional Travel and Tourism Caucus for the U.S. House of Representatives spread her influence nationwide.

Like June, today's pacesetting baby boomer allows the beauty of God to rest upon her and radiates multicolored beams of God's love to her world. With the excitement of the new life of Jesus living inside you, it is time to shine!

• QUESTIONS FOR IMMEDIATE APPLICATION •

1 What would you say is the relationship between aging and the spiritual life?
2. What are you currently doing to cultivate your spirituality? What would you like to do?
3. When have you experienced spiritual empowerment, what has helped you cope with issues of aging?

• FAVORITE SCRIPTURE PASSAGES ON AGING •

Children's children are a crown to the aged, and parents are the pride of their children. (Proverbs 17:6 NIV)

Do not forget my teaching, but let your heart keep my commandments; for length of days and years of life, and peace they will add to you. (Proverbs 3:1–2)

The righteous will flourish like the palm tree....Planted in the house of the LORD, they will flourish in the courts of our God. They will still yield fruit in old age; they shall be full of sap and very green. (Psalm 92:12–14)

I will fulfill the number of your days. (Exodus 23:26)

Strength and dignity are her clothing, and she smiles at the future. (Proverbs 31:25)

Even to your old age, I shall be the same, and even to your graying years I shall bear you! I have done it, and I shall carry you; and I shall bear you, and I shall deliver you.

(Isaiah 46:4)

For I know the plans that I have for you...plans for welfare and not for calamity to give you a future and a hope.

(Jeremiah 29:11)

Gray hair is a crown of splendor; it is attained by a righteous life. (Proverbs 16:31 NIV)

He has made everything beautiful in its time.

(Ecclesiastes 3:11 NIV)

A jubilee shall that fiftieth year be. (Leviticus 25:11 KJV)

AGING SUCCESSFULLY: ATTITUDE #3

A personal relationship with Jesus Christ is the life preserver that will save us from sinking into the sea of aging and empower us to experience the sparkling, jewellike beauty of being God's ageless woman.

CHAPTER 4

HERITAGE, HAPPINESS, AND HOPE IN MIDLIFE: SHAPING OUR SPIRITUAL LIVES

"Those of us who have tasted from the sweet spring of intimacy with God will never again be satisfied with lapping from earth's polluted pools."

—Jamie Buckingham

"Be still, and know that I am God."

—Psalm 46:10 (NIV)

When I was 37 years old, my family doctor broke the news: I was pregnant. I knew my organized, well-ordered life with my husband and two beautiful teenagers would end after nine months had passed. My spirit was disquieted within me.

• THE IMPORTANCE OF DAILY QUIET TIME •

Each morning after our teenagers had swirled off to school in clouds of panic, perfume, and aftershave, and after my husband had rushed to work, I breathed deeply and enjoyed what I called my quiet time. I would take this time to be intimate with my God. I talked to Him, listened to Him, read His Word, and allowed the Holy Spirit to direct me in setting priorities and making goals.

As I sat in the presence of the Lord, my heart and mind anxious and unsettled, He allowed me to envision a big, silver fish. When the fish was taken out of the water and put on the ground, it flopped and flipped. I recognized this as my attitude toward my upcoming new lifestyle—bottles, diapers, and sleepless nights. Removed from my normal, well-ordered element, I would thrash about restlessly.

Then, in my mind's eye, I saw the big, silver fish slip back into the clear, cool water and glide gracefully away.

With this vision, I knew God had me in the right element, in the center of His perfect will. I sensed that He wanted me to relax and be joyful in Him, just as that fish relaxed and was joyful in the clear water. Knowing that God was in charge and capable of caring for all the changes ahead helped me find peace with my pregnancy.

After nine months, I delivered a healthy baby boy. Jay recently graduated from college and has always brought joy to everyone around him, confirming God's wisdom in planning my late-in-life pregnancy. For me, staying in touch with God enabled me to find His plan and the peace that goes with it. Regular quiet times of intimacy with God keep life on God's track, so that aging becomes a positive instead of a negative. God's changelessness helps us face the future and aging's ensuing changes with courage. (See James 1:17.)

A daily time alone with God propels us into eternal and universal living. It gives us divine personal power. Just as handsome antique furniture gleams with character and value, so with God does life become richer and mellower with age, enhancing our character.

Don't allow the toils and cares of the day to rob you of sweet fellowship with your Creator. A daily quiet time keeps us in touch with God and with ourselves, and guides each moment. It keeps us from having a fat life and an emaciated soul.

Solitude

One component of a quiet time is solitude. Life can become extremely complicated and busy! "Busyness lends a false sense of importance to our days," writes Jane Rubietta, one of my dearest friends, in *Quiet Places: A Woman's Guide to Personal Retreat.* "If we're busy, we must be valuable....This perpetual churning thinly covers the lack of meaning, shielding us from our fear of nothingness. It also substitutes for waiting on God....The only antidote I have found to busyness is solitude."[1]

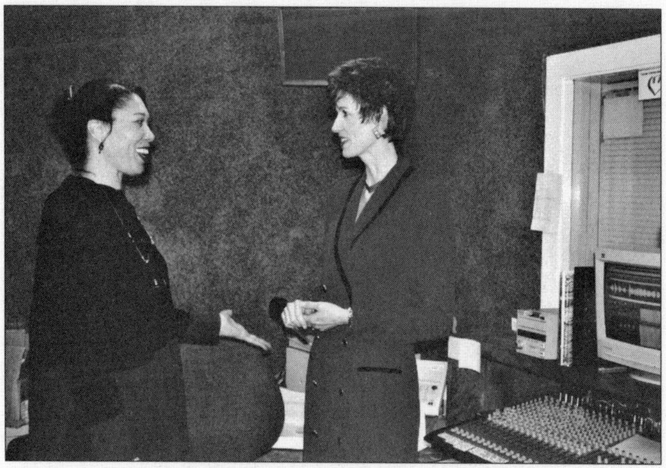

Jane Rubietta (right) on a live talk show,
Saahara Glaude's WYDE-VIEW, in Birmingham, Alabama

Jane, a remarkable woman of God, says that in solitude, we can shed our mask of busyness and begin to find real rest and renewed meaning in God. Solitude is a treasured time to converse with God, find rest and solace in His bosom, be lifted to the weightlessness of His Spirit, and seek His guidance.

Here are several simple steps to insure some time of quiet:

1. Find a private, comfortable, cheerful place for meditation.
2. Decide the time of day that fits your lifestyle, preferably when you are most alert. This time can be flexible and can even be spread throughout the day.
3. Collect the necessary tools: your favorite translation of the Bible or perhaps a parallel Bible with several different translations lined up alongside each other; a pen and a journal for recording thoughts, prayers, answered prayers, and dreams; devotional books and a Bible concordance to help you dig nuggets of gold from God's Word for your aging and improving life; and a personal planning calendar. Then, do it!

Meeting the Master face-to-face is life changing! Perceiving God's holiness, perfection, love, and majesty explodes mature living into heights never before experienced in life!

As you pray, talk to God as an intimate friend. Remember that good friends not only talk but also listen, yet listening to God is often overlooked in our haste to move on. God speaks to our minds through His Word, the Scriptures. "*My sheep hear my voice*," says Jesus, "*and I know them, and they follow me*" (John 10:27 KJV).

J. I. Packer, in *Knowing God*, says, "God's Word is His almighty speech. God's Spirit is His almighty breath."[2] As we draw near to God during our quiet time, we begin to understand how Moses must have felt when he drew near the burning bush. (See Exodus 3.) A quiet time is "holy ground."

Knowing God, and knowing that the Bible is the primary authority and power for our lives, gives us confidence to live the latter half of our lives victoriously. We are foolish if we choose anything less than God. If we cheat ourselves out of the miracle of intimacy with Him, we deprive ourselves of the abundant life. Old age can be viewed as a thief that "*comes only to steal, and kill, and destroy,*" but Jesus comes "*that* [we] *might have life, and might have it abundantly*" (John 10:10).

The Benefits of Quiet Time

Time spent alone with God reaps wonderful rewards!

> *"Because he loves me,"* says the LORD, *"I will rescue him; I will protect him, for he acknowledges my name. He will call on me, and I will answer him; I will be with him in trouble, I will deliver him and honor him. With long life I will satisfy him and show him my salvation."* (Psalm 91:14–16 NIV)

Amazingly, this time of loving God and being loved in return overflows as service in our lives, setting our hearts free and giving us a weightless spirit like that of the monarch butterfly. When aging and gravity would pull us down, God lifts us up!

Flowing through us, as well, will be God's energizing power. "*They go from strength to strength, till each appears before God in Zion*" (Psalm 84:7 NIV). What a mystery. When we give God even a snippet of our time, He exchanges our feeble and finite energy for His unlimited strength.

Loving God reaps rewards for us physically, as well. Researchers at the University of Texas analyzed surveys from 12,000 American adults. Results showed that day-to-day involvement in a religious community...

> seemed to extend the lives of congregants by about seven years. The results were even stronger for African Americans. People who reported attending religious services

more than once a week lived, on average, 14 years longer than those who said they never attend.[3]

Those who did not attend worship services, "were much more likely to have died, and were several times as likely to have succumbed to infectious diseases, diabetes, or respiratory illness."[4] It seems there are many reasons for "*not forsaking the assembling of ourselves together*" (Hebrews 10:25 KJV).

Just off of my bedroom patio grows a beautiful oak tree, strong and straight. As the vast, sprawling root system goes deep into the fertile soil, the oak tree on top of the ground grows tall and broad, spreading its branches far into the air.

An aging Christian whose inner life is growing deep into the Spirit of God will display a strong, straight, powerful outer life. The nutrients of a clean heart, a God-centered life, and a simple faith will cause the roots of prayer, Bible study, and revelation to produce a mighty oak in you.

The prophet Isaiah calls us trees of righteousness, the planting of the Lord, that He might be glorified. (See Isaiah 61:3.)

• HOW TO DRAW CLOSE TO GOD •

For a number of years, I was privileged to sing with the magnificent Albertville, Alabama, First Baptist Choir. Singing at church every Sunday brought me closer to God. One morning, the energizing, rhythmic offertory entranced me. Dale Cotton, our pianist, presided over the ivory keys of the baby grand piano. As her fingers flew, the melody of "His Eye Is on the Sparrow" brought the lyrics to mind. At the sound of my favorite hymn, tears of joy filled my eyes. If God loves a sparrow that much, how He must treasure us! I am learning to let my heart rest in God's hand like a bird in a nest.

God's Word tells us, "*But it is good for me to draw near to God: I have put my trust in the Lord* GOD, *that I may declare all thy works*" (Psalm 73:28 KJV). Think about it! We can trust someone only if we know him well, and we come to know God well in several ways.

One sure way to draw near to God is to read the Bible. When asked, "How do you encounter God?" singer and author Pat Boone responded,

> Most mornings, after my physical and spiritual exercises, I try to sit down and let Him speak to me out of His Word, the Bible....I let the psalmist David "prime my pump," and from there I usually move into specific prayer, asking God to help me and others who have particular needs.

Without being grounded in God's Word, we run the risk of trusting the wrong voice. By reading the Scriptures, we balance out the relationship, not merely giving God our list of needs, demands, and requests but listening to Him speak through the Bible.

A second way to draw near to God is to think about Him. Contemplating His divinity humbles us, at the same time expanding our thinking.

God knows when we talk and think about Him.

> *Then they that feared the* LORD *spake often one to another: and the* LORD *hearkened, and heard it, and a book of remembrance was written before him for them that feared the* LORD, *and that thought upon his name. And they shall be mine, saith the* LORD *of hosts, in that day when I make up my jewels; and I will spare them, as a man spareth his own son that serveth him.* (Malachi 3:16–17 KJV)

Several other practices lead us closer to God: knowing His character, observing His presence, keeping away from sin and praising God and worshiping God.

• GETTING TO KNOW THE CHARACTER OF GOD •

As we draw near to God, we discover incredible truths about His character.

God Loves Us

Perhaps the most amazing of all is that God is loving. He loves us, and has loved us from our mother's womb.

> *My frame was not hidden from you when I was made in the secret place. When I was woven together in the depths of the earth, your eyes saw my unformed body. All the days ordained for me were written in your book before one of them came to be.*
> (Psalm 139:15–16 NIV)

He loves us so much that He will take care of all that concerns us. *"The LORD will perfect that which concerneth me: thy mercy, O LORD, endureth for ever: forsake not the works of thine own hands"* (Psalm 138:8 KJV). If this verse doesn't erase your worry wrinkles, nothing will! In addition, our full potential will be released when we draw close to someone who loves us unconditionally.

God Is Omnipotent

My friend June reminds me of a second characteristic of God. Her ageless life and great achievements might make another puffed up and proud, but when I asked her how she managed her responsibilities as sales director of Lake Guntersville State Lodge, as well as her appointment by Congressman Tom Bevill to the advisory board of the Congressional Travel and Tourism

Caucus for the U.S. House of Representatives, her million-dollar smile shone, and she said, "Without the almighty power behind us, we would be nothing!" June's intimate relationship with Jesus Christ affirmed my belief that God is not just a mystical figure somewhere out in the universe. He is real, and He has all power.

Theologians call this trait *omnipotence*. We see this truth in Scripture, time and again: *"For with God nothing shall be impossible"* (Luke 1:37 KJV). God, our omnipotent Father, made you and me. He understands what makes each of us tick and knows more about us than we know about ourselves. He knows our deepest fears and our most secret dreams, and He is able to bring about His amazing will for each of us.

God Is Omnipresent

Several years ago, this powerful God gave me the opportunity to travel with a tour group to the Holy Land. Israel was a hot spot at that time because a Christian was responsible for shooting several Muslims at the Wailing Wall. God demonstrated His power in my own soul when He surrounded me with perfect peace about entering into troubled Jerusalem. Even while powerfully protecting my spirit, God demonstrated another great truth about Himself: His ability to be everywhere at once (omnipresence).

When I prayed about my concerns over traveling overseas without my husband and ever-expanding family of three children, two children-in-law, and five lovely granddaughters, God whispered into my heart, *I am everywhere. I can take care of you just as easily in Israel as in Albertville, Alabama. And I can take care of your loved ones, as well.* After receiving this reassurance, I traveled in quiet peace. Faith in God is an oasis of peace, even when surrounded by the swirling sands of conflict and the passing of time.

The trip to the Holy Land was mind expanding and spiritually rewarding. After this experience, my life exploded with energy as the sense of God's continual presence lodged in my heart. The Scriptures confirm this, as well:

> *Acknowledge and take to heart this day that the* Lord *is God in heaven above and on the earth below. There is no other. Keep His decrees and commands, which I am giving you today, so that it may go well with you and your children after you and that you may live long in the land the* Lord *your God gives you for all time.* (Deuteronomy 4:39–40 NIV)

What a promise! God's omnipresence makes life an adventure with love. The whole universe is filled with His presence. This fact gives me much faith, whether I'm praying for someone on the other side of the globe or traveling out of my natural element—and up in the air.

Flying to Russia with a group of people in the food industry, I felt my insides short circuit as fear muddled my mind. All the what-ifs of flying—What if we crash? What if we're shot out of the air? What if there's a hostage situation or a medical crisis?—constricted my heart until I could barely breathe. Finally, God managed to gather me to Himself, much like a gentle father would soothe a terrified child by pulling her into his arms, and I realized that God is with me in the air as well as on the ground. He's not limited by space!

The lyrics to a childhood song reminded me, "He is big enough to rule the universe but small enough to live in my heart." God's ubiquitous presence will illuminate our minds to the growing range of possibilities in mature living.

God Is Omniscient

Knowing that God has all knowledge (omniscience) also expands our horizons.

Corrie ten Boom, a Christian who harbored Jews in her home during World War II, was arrested along with the rest of her family by the Nazis and sent to a concentration camp. She and one sister survived the horrendous experience full of strength and faith, knowing that God was in charge of their lives and fully aware of every intimate detail. God so strengthened Corrie that she circled the world, sharing a message of faith and love and forgiveness. In her total surrender to Christ, she depended upon Him rather than her circumstances for her joy.

There is nothing in our lives that God does not both know about and allow. This knowledge makes a timeless woman sparkle with optimism! Knowing Jehovah God is sovereign gives the ageless woman confidence and security.

> *I am God, and there is no other; I am God, and there is none like me. I make known the end from the beginning, from ancient times, what is still to come. I say: My purpose will stand, and I will do all that I please....What I have said, that will I bring about; what I have planned, that will I do. Listen to me, you stubborn-hearted, you who are now far from my righteousness. I am bringing my righteousness near, it is not far away; and my salvation will not be delayed. I will grant salvation to Zion, my splendor to Israel.* (Isaiah 46:9–13 NIV)

God Is Triune

The more we know about God, the more incredible and well planned our lives seem to be! In perfect wisdom, God knew we would need lifelong parenting, and so calls Himself our Father.

"O Lord, *you are our Father. We are the clay, you are the potter; we are all the work of your hand"* (Isaiah 64:8 NIV). This is the first aspect of what Christians have come to call the Trinity: God the Father, God the Son, and God the Holy Spirit. In Christ we have God the Son. *"Jesus said...'I am the way, and the truth, and the life; no one comes to the Father, but through Me'"* (John 14:6). And then, before Jesus ascended into heaven to sit at the right hand of the heavenly Father, He said, *"But you shall receive power when the Holy Spirit has come upon you"* (Acts 1:8). He had comforted His followers about His own leaving by saying, *"And I will ask the Father, and He will give you another Helper, that He may be with you forever; that is the Spirit of truth....I will not leave you as orphans; I will come to you"* (John 14:16–18).

This same Spirit guides our lives, comforts us, and gives us power! What a miracle! All eternity is held in one moment of God's presence. Our only response can be one of praise.

• PRAISING GOD •

Knowing and praising God makes the 50-plus woman delightfully different. Praise brings enormous benefits. Praise is an age-buster, perhaps the greatest beauty secret of all time. Praise lifts our face, our faith, our spirit, our attitude, and even our step! Praise defies the natural tendency to move downward, both in firmness and in feature—it puts a smile on our face and laughter in our heart.

One benefit of praising God is exchanging a spirit of heaviness for a garment of praise. The prophet Isaiah gives us the message that Jesus came...

> *to appoint unto them that mourn in Zion, to give unto them beauty for ashes, the oil of joy for mourning, the garment of praise for the spirit of heaviness; that they might be called trees*

> *of righteousness, the planting of the LORD, that he might be glorified.* (Isaiah 61:3 KJV)

Unwavering confidence in God leads to a spontaneous attitude of gratitude and praise, whatever the circumstances. Paul E. Billheimer said, "Praise is the spark plug of faith."[4] We can pray with the psalmist, "*Praise be to the LORD God, the God of Israel, who alone does marvelous deeds. Praise be to his glorious name forever; may the whole earth be filled with his glory. Amen and Amen*" (Psalm 72:18–19 NIV).

"Affirmation is vital in intimate relationships, and none more so than in our relationship with the Lord. The Scriptures call forth praise from the people for the person of God," writes Jane Rubietta in her book *Quiet Places*.[5] Thus, when we praise God, we are exulting in His characteristics, such as His steadfast love, quick forgiveness, holiness, knowledge, presence, and power. We also praise God when we thank Him for His mighty activity in our lives, for working behind the scenes, tirelessly, to assure that all things work together for each of us. Bringing all these praises to mind lifts us up to heaven!

Praise Draws Us Close to God

Praise the Lord! Praise puts us in the arena of God's presence. Sin, on the other hand, separates us from God.

> *And the leper in whom the plague is, his clothes shall be rent, and his head bare, and he shall put a covering upon his upper lip, and shall cry, Unclean, unclean. All the days wherein the plague shall be in him he shall be defiled; he is unclean; he shall dwell alone; without the camp shall his habitation be.*
> (Leviticus 13:45–46 KJV)

The word *leper* struck terror in the hearts of the Israelites for two reasons. First, the person who had leprosy became an outcast and was forced to leave his home, family, friends, and place of worship to live outside the camp. When anyone went near, the leper had to cry out, "Unclean! Unclean!" But perhaps the biggest reason leprosy was so feared was that there was no known cure for it, and thus it led to permanent isolation, from loved ones as well as from God.

Leprosy is symbolic of how horrible sin is. Sin destroys the joy of life and, if it continues, will eventually lead to the ruin of both body and soul. The leper's separation from the place of sacrifice and worship illustrates how sin separates us from the presence of God.

> *Listen now! The Lord isn't too weak to save you. And He isn't getting deaf! He can hear you when you call! But the trouble is that your sins have cut you off from God. Because of sin he has turned his face away from you and will not listen anymore.*
> (Isaiah 59:1–2 TLB)

Some of the darkest times of life are when we sin and cut ourselves off from God. God does not move, but we move away from Him when we sin. However, focusing on the good news of Jesus Christ, we have the power to turn those dark times into light.

Jesus Christ, God's Son, was born on this earth, lived a perfect life, and was crucified and buried; on the third day, He arose from the dead. He ascended into heaven and now sits at the right hand of God, the Father, interceding for you and me. He runs interference for us, convicting our hearts on earth and pleading for us before God in heaven.

Beautifully, though, we are assured of God's positive response to our confession of sin.

"God delights to pour forgiveness into that hollowness created by confession, generating a spilling of praise," writes Jane Rubietta in *Still Waters: Finding the Place Where God Restores Your Soul.*[6] First John 1:9 says, "*If we confess our sins, he is faithful and just to forgive us our sins, and to cleanse us from all unrighteousness*" (KJV).

Praise Gives Us Hope

Praising God leads us into places of hope! Let no discouragement or weariness cause you to turn loose the rope of hope, which is in Christ Jesus. "*The LORD is my portion, saith my soul; therefore will I hope in him*" (Lamentations 3:24 KJV).

However, as Tyne Daly has said, hope is a muscle, and muscles grow by working them out. Thankfully, the muscle of hope grows simply by loving God more and more. So, crawl up into His lap and allow Him to wrap His warm arms of love around you. Like lovers, spend quality time together, expanding that love.

• QUESTIONS FOR IMMEDIATE APPLICATION •

1. In a short paragraph, share how you currently cultivate your relationship with God in a daily time of quiet and why it is special to you. If you are not currently having a quiet time, write out a plan for practicing quiet time in the future.
2. List four ways you will draw close to God.
3. What will give you wings to fly through your maturing life with joy?

• TOP TEN FAVORITE HAPPINESS STRATEGIES •

1. Remember Solomon's words: "*There is nothing better for them than to rejoice and to do good in one's lifetime*" (Ecclesiastes 3:12).

2. Another axiom to live by: "As you think in your heart, so are you." (See Proverbs 23:7.)
3. Positive thoughts make positive lives.
4. Have a plan. Know what makes you happy. Do it.
5. When your mood swings down, start moving.
6. Dwell on positive things. "*Whatever is true, whatever is honorable, whatever is right, whatever is pure, whatever is lovely, whatever is of good repute, if there is any excellence and if anything worthy of praise, let your mind dwell on these things*" (Philippians 4:8).
7. Practice thanksgiving and praise.
8. Journaling has medical benefits and makes room for happiness by moving the unhappiness to the outside. "A *tranquil heart is life to the body*" (Proverbs 14:30).
9. Dance. King David did. (See 2 Samuel 6:14.) Dance in your heart, in your kitchen, in your attitude, in your garden....
10. Smile. It changes the way you see the world—and the way the world sees you.

AGING SUCCESSFULLY: ATTITUDE #4

Knowing God through a daily time of quiet intimacy propels our life into universal and eternal living. It gives us wings to fly through our maturing life.

CHAPTER 5

COURAGEOUS AGING: SHAPING AND CHANGING THE FUTURE

"A person doesn't spring into existence at the age of 50; there are years of preparation, which God uses in ways we may never know."[1]

—Corrie ten Boom

"Strength and dignity are her clothing, and she smiles at the future."

—Proverbs 31:25

The silk flowed luxuriously around me as I walked toward the large, beautifully draped living room window and gazed out upon the spacious, well-groomed lawn, which highlighted the sharp contrast between my past and my present. In the house where I grew up, on a cotton farm, our primary source of entertainment was the huge radio in our living room. We danced to the music it produced, huddled around to hear the news programs, and gasped at the soap operas. After listening to a newscast one morning, my beautiful, auburn-haired mother sent me to the back 40 acres, where my dad was tilling the land with two horses pulling a turning plow.

Carrying earth-shattering good news and some refreshing, cold water, I walked barefoot in the freshly plowed ground, my legs sinking almost to my knees in the warm dirt, as I made my way slowly to my dad. Even from a distance, his big, expressive green eyes shot beams of love my way.

With sweat dripping from his chin and a wide grin stretched across his tanned, young face, he watched my halting progress. I waited till the water had revived him, then spilled my news: "The war is over! World War II is over!" He hooped and hollered, grabbed me up, crushed me to his damp chest, and spun me around in the pungent dirt.

Working land that wasn't our own and putting aside money to buy a patch of ground for our home, cutting down trees and sawing our own lumber for the little, four-room house in the middle of the potato patch, building the home ourselves in the few spare hours available each day—that was our life.

But scratching out an existence could not squelch my dreams; rather, I believe it compelled me to reach and stretch and work hard to achieve those dreams. I would not be writing, speaking, and investing in the lives of others had I not learned the power of hard work and the importance of dreams.

• FIRST THINGS FIRST •

Before dreaming big, however, as women approaching the years of fabulous 50 and beyond, we have to recognize our losses. Life is full of them, especially as we age, and it's vital to acknowledge those losses in order to honor the process of life. Grief is an appropriate emotion to encounter as we age. We *have* lost some things, things even more vital than youth in this culture that worships it. Noticing is not vanity; it is a reality check, and it's imperative to finding our focus after the age of 50.

Creating a list of personal losses may help each of us grieve, so that we may then move on. Some possibilities include the loss of loved ones, loss of a beloved home, or personal losses of health, agility, body function, and even body parts.[2]

Other losses may be more subtle and less obvious to the casual observer of life. Loss may look like disappointment, broken dreams, disillusionment with our relationships or with the way we've fulfilled our chosen roles of wife, mother, friend, employee, and so forth. Losses may include mistakes which have cost us, or another, greatly.

Freedom to grieve these losses—to acknowledge them and say, "I am sad about this aspect of life or love"—grants us the ability to heal and then ultimately refocus our lives. It is important to learn how to shift our focus from what we have lost to who we are becoming and to how we will impact the world in our remaining years.

• PLANNING FOR THE FUTURE •

All the longevity in the world, all the medical tricks of the trade, will not assure a high quality of life. The question we must now answer is not how to live longer, not how to look good while living longer, but what we will live for.

In answering that basic question, we find not only the motivation to live longer but also the energy and passion to care for our bodies through a healthy diet, exercise, and appropriate self-care. This motivation gives us the energy to live, to live well, and to live long.

"Aging well takes some planning. It's so easy to lose focus, fail to stretch for the best life has to offer, and end life full of regrets," writes Valerie Bell.[3]

To plan for the future—not necessarily *where* we will live out our remaining years but *how* we will live them—we must, as

Olympia Dukakis says, take time to evaluate, question, and find anew our reason to go on.[4]

Figuring out our purpose for the next 30 to 50 years is crucial. As Joan Rivers put it, "What so many...seniors miss...is a sense of *purpose*, which is essential at *every* age. You've got to have a better reason to get up in the morning than to plan your lunch."[5]

Midlife is a time when we expand our focus from the tiny nucleus of self and family and begin giving back. Whether this is through paid work or through volunteering is less important than the actual investment of our passion and energy into others. Eleanor Roosevelt said, "When you cease to make a contribution, you begin to die." Finding out how to invest in others' lives will give us renewed reasons to feel better and live longer.

Our life purpose must extend beyond our own limited number of years and impact another generation.

• DREAM ON •

One of our greatest challenges as human beings is to live life without regret. Now is a chance to rethink the future, to listen to that still, small voice that has, from time to time, whispered a dream to your heart. Is there a rustling in your soul, urging you, "There's something more"? What might some of those long-buried dreams be?

The Scriptures remind us of the importance of listening to those dreams.

> *And it shall come to pass afterward, that I will pour out my spirit upon all flesh; and your sons and your daughters shall prophesy, your old men shall dream dreams, your young men shall see visions.* (Joel 2:28 KJV)

Thomas Kinkade writes:

> When God comes near, wonderful things begin to happen. A dull people become visionary. The timid are given new courage. Old men, who felt that life had passed them by, suddenly feel that God is making them useful once again....But perhaps the greatest gift of all is vision. When we feel the force of some new dream welling up within us, we are most alive.[6]

Age is no barrier to either dreaming or achieving. Countless models have shown us the way. Peter Mark Roget was first a doctor in the 1800s; only after retiring at the age of 61 did he begin to work on the first edition of his *Thesaurus.* It took him 12 years; little did he know that his "little tool" would survive into the next millennium!

Grandma Moses started painting at age 80. She created 25 percent of her famous paintings as a centenarian. "Michaelangelo did some of his best painting when past eighty; Goethe wrote when past eighty; Edison was still inventing at ninety-two. Frank Lloyd Wright at ninety was considered the most creative architect; Shaw was still writing plays at ninety."[7] Furthermore, hardship is no inhibitor of dreaming and achievement:

> When a man is determined, what can stop him? Cripple him and you have a Sir Walter Scott. Put him in a prison cell and you have a John Bunyan. Bury him in the snows of Valley Forge and you have a George Washington. Have him born in abject poverty and you have a Lincoln. Put him in the grease pit of a locomotive roundhouse and you have a Walter P. Chrysler. Make him second fiddle in an obscure South African orchestra and you have a Toscanini. The hardships of life are sent not...to crush, but to challenge.[8]

So, what are the dreams tugging at the sleeve of your heart right now? Jan Karon, who did not even graduate from high school, faced her dreams after working her way up in an advertising firm. She quit her job in her 40s and began writing books—and is now the best-selling author of the Mitford series. Perhaps your dream is to take a different job or pursue further schooling, to sell the farm (or buy a farm!), to start your own business, to backpack in the Andes, or to learn to dance or to swim or to speak a different language. Interestingly enough, pursing our dreams will benefit our health, as well:

> Our bodies are designed to function best when we're involved in activities and work that feel exactly right to us. Our health is enhanced when we engage in deeply creative work that is satisfying to *us*—not just because it pleases our boss, husband, or mother. This work can range from gardening to computer programming to welding.[9]

Whatever items compose your list, be done with the excuses. We can no longer blame our past, our parents, or our imperfections. Ladies, it's time to stop simmering and start cooking!

• REDEFINING OUR WORK •

As we consider our dreams and examine our purpose, we must also recognize that older people are living healthier, and thus living longer, and may need to work for health, fulfillment, and monetary needs alike. Work may be an economic necessity for many 50-plus people, but that doesn't mean that our work must be drudgery. We needn't become obsolete in the job market simply because we are technologically behind.

Marie, for example, continues to take computer courses at night, honing her knowledge of the instrument that became a personal tool long after her own children had graduated from college. Now, at age 63, she finds accounting mistakes made by younger employees with their master's degree. She has kept herself viable and employed long after many have given up the race. She keeps herself fit and active, covers the gray hair and cuts it becomingly, and has edged many a younger person out of the running for her job because she isn't afraid to learn new skills. Her maturity and quiet wisdom have earned her respect in a youthful market.

The trend of women working—and staying employed into their later years—has impacted the U.S. economy. In the last eight years, the number of female-owned businesses has increased 180 percent—while ownership of small business increased just 12 percent! Thirty-eight percent of all businesses in America are now owned by women, generating nearly four trillion dollars in revenue a year.[10]

Volunteer

The after-50 set makes up the ranks of the largest volunteer base ever in America. From soup kitchens to church nurseries, from tutoring to teaching in graduate schools, seniors are learning that there is more to life than club-hopping and culture.

When Linda turned 50, she decided to figure out her purpose in life. Her church has a program for mothers called MOPS (Mothers of Preschoolers), and Linda, remembering how difficult those years could be, decided to volunteer as a mentor. In the process of finding herself, she has discovered great joy in listening to and mentoring younger mothers.

At age 45, Arlene Shipley and her husband became the foster parents of a nine-year-old girl who had been sexually abused and was dying from the effects of AIDS. Little Tashia lived two years, and after her death, Arlene started up

AngelAID, "a volunteer- and donation-based foundation in Jacksonville, Florida, providing free medical treatment, activities, and guidance for children and families who fall between the cracks of government programs." Now, six years later, Arlene oversees a staff of volunteers and handles a caseload of more than 2,000 children.[11]

For 15 years, another volunteer named Molly, now 86, has delivered food to "older people" who are too weak to leave their apartments. She knows "that life at its best is giving and worrying about someone besides yourself."[12]

This is compassion in action, and it's happening across the continent in record numbers. Opportunities abound, even for those who long to travel.[13] Church denominations around the world are beginning to organize groups that cater to the "leisure set," allowing volunteers to travel as well as give back. Short-term missions are another possibility for the senior who desires to see the world and change it, too.

Kay, for example, wanted to give back to the youth, and so, at age 58, she volunteered to chaperone a trip to Appalachia. For seven days, she sweat, laughed, and worked like crazy with a bunch of high schoolers. "It was the best week of my life," she says, still laughing. She proudly displays a picture of herself and her group in front of the home they helped refurbish. She is covered with dirt and wearing an enormous smile.

Studies are finding that involvement in volunteering helps others and helps the volunteer! Not only is this a way to cope with loss, volunteering keeps our minds stretching and vital, keeps our focus broader than ourselves, and helps us live longer.

> In 1986, the University of Michigan surveyed 1,211 adults over age 65 (mostly retirees) and found that about 35 percent regularly donated time to a church, charity,

> or other organization. Over the next eight years the scientists compared the well-being of the community helpers with that of the others. Remarkably, volunteering seemed to delay death, even when differences in the two groups' health, income, and number of weekly social interactions were factored out. People giving up to 40 hours a year to one cause were 40 percent more likely than non-volunteers to be alive at the study's end.[14]

If our lives don't make a difference, what difference does it make if we have our health?

Just Plain Fun Is Fine

Along with giving to the next generation out of the storehouses of wisdom and experience we've accumulated, it's important to remember that fun is fine! Cruise lines are focusing on the retiring market by offering affordable packages to "new" elders who are aging with vigor, power, and style.

The recent retiree may be cruising the "age wave" on a fun ship. The 50-plus Americans migrating up the lifeline are in charge of 70 percent of the net worth in the United States, according to Dr. Ken Dychtwald, author of *Age Wave*. With that in mind, retirement in the new millennium may be a new beginning when dreams come true for the average retiree.

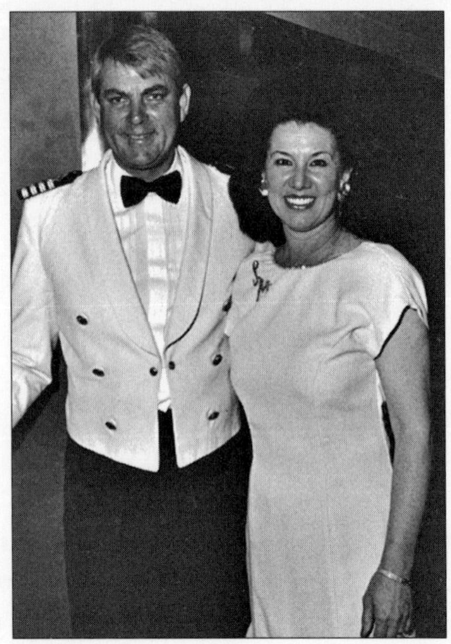

Shirley with the captain of M/S Sunward II,
Norwegian Caribbean Cruise Lines

My own experience cruising the Caribbean made me feel fabulous, fit, and feisty, with an indefatigable spirit and unrestricted exuberance. The mystique of a new adventure, mysterious beauty of the sea, sensational sun, sumptuous food, and spirit of camaraderie made the cruise a time to remember. As I mature, I find I prefer valuable experiences more than valuable things.

I learned how enamored I am of mornings on the sea. On the ocean, my thoughts flow easily. The magnificent rising and falling waves of the vast ocean covering 70 percent of this great earth always makes me feel close to God.

It also inspired me to write poetry. Sitting on the deck of the cruise ship waiting for sunrise after a vigorous walk, I watched in hushed expectancy. Feeling God's presence, I wrote the following poem as the sun popped over the horizon, spilling gorgeous hues of red, orange, and yellow into the sky.

"SUNRISE ON THE AZURE SEA"

by Shirley W. Mitchell

The seething ocean waves
of the Atlantic
slapped the morning
with splashes of delight!

The sea gulls flapped
their wings wildly,
anticipating the ending
of the night.

Then that glorious
ball of fire
popped over the horizon,
embracing the morning with pure delight.

The waves, the seagulls, and I
felt God's presence
as He kissed the morning
with a silent burst of golden light.

• FREE TO GIVE, FREE TO LIVE •

After 50, we find the joy of giving back, pouring into others, and returning and serving out of the rich storehouse of the knowledge and experience we have gained. Life after 50 is not, after all, one long, aimless, self-centered pursuit of pleasure and passion but a time when we are free to give. Thus, we find the fullness, focus, and value of the second half of life. Daring to dream larger than ourselves and living for others leaves a legacy of hope, love, and meaning.

• QUESTIONS FOR IMMEDIATE APPLICATION •

1. Create your own list of personal losses; grieve, and then move on into creative living. To maximize the time, figure out what you have learned from your hardships.
2. List three dreams, and three ways you will follow your dreams.
3. List ways you will give from the rich storehouse of knowledge and experience you have gained over 50 years of living.

• "FOCUS ON THE FUTURE" STRATEGIES •

1. If you could do anything and go anywhere, what and where would that be?
2. Everyone should volunteer somewhere. It's good food for the soul to give our best for free! Where would your gifts and expertise best be put to use?
3. Keep stretching–body, mind, and spirit.
4. Adopt this prayer of King David: *"Even when I am old and gray, O God, do not forsake me, until I declare Thy strength to this generation, Thy power to all who are to come"* (Psalm 71:18).
5. Dare to dream. Dream big, dream small–just dream! We minimize God's power and our own potential when we don't dream.
6. List the legacy you want to leave behind. What do you want people to say about you when you die?
7. Write down the ways you'd like to impact the next generation.
8. Brainstorm areas for self-improvement.

9. Surround yourself with people who surpass your abilities; it will not only keep you humble but also help you to grow.
10. List your goals and objectives for the second half of your life. Dare to get involved, to love, and to live fully.

AGING SUCCESSFULLY: ATTITUDE #5

I will choose to live fully after 50, dreaming new dreams and investing my energies in others.

CHAPTER 6

FAMILY AND FRIENDS AFTER 50

"The years seem to rush by now, and I think of death as a fast-approaching end of a journey. Double and treble the reason for...loving while it is day."

—George Eliot, in a letter, 1861

"Let us consider how to stimulate one another to love and good deeds...encouraging one another; and all the more as you see the day drawing near."

—Hebrews 10:24–25

Warm, happy laughter, small children's sweet voices, and commotion filled the air as the people I loved crowded into the restaurant. Four banquet tables that had been pushed together disappeared under plates filled with food. I pressed my hand to my chest, feeling as though my heart would burst. Love for my children, grandchildren, and best friends filled me up and brought tears to my eyes. I could not stop smiling as I drank in the beauty of the moment.

Relationships are life-giving, and we must seize every opportunity to devote ourselves to giving life in our relationships! Study after study shows the impact of having meaningful, supportive community: we'll live longer and enjoy better health if we are involved in lives outside of our own. One study found the following:

> People with many ties (marriage, close friendships, extended families, church membership, or group associations) had a far lower mortality rate than those who lacked quality or depth in their social support systems.[1]

Another study "indicated that men in their fifties, at high risk because of a low social and economic status, but who score high on an index of social networks, lived far longer than high status men with low social network scores."[2] Social isolation can cause emotional, mental, and physical deterioration.

> The aging need opportunities for a continuation of the creative work which, fundamentally, is essential to any significant human experience. It is not enough to kill time with what are called hobbies, to sit about, even in the sunshine and in the company of other aging people, doing nothing more than waiting for death. The aging must be given opportunity to continue, as long as there is breath within them, to serve the people and purpose, the causes, institutions, and enterprises which gave meaning to the whole course of their lives.[3]

• LIFE-GIVING RELATIONSHIPS •

Relationships give our lives depth, breadth, and a reason for living well. Our first relationship, one we may not always consider, is our relationship with ourselves. As we become self-aware, understanding the emotions we are feeling and our motives for acting, owning, and being broken by those feelings and motives, we become a *safe* place for others—nonjudgmental, accepting, and loving. This frees us up to be involved more deeply in the lives of others, starting with our immediate family members.

Your Husband

Whether you've been married to the man of your dreams for many years or for only a few, mature marriage has the possibility of being warm and exciting, like a sunbath on the deck of a luxury cruise ship. Think of all the learning and adjusting that has gone into creating a lasting marriage—this is a gift to be treasured while aging together. Savoring memories while creating new ones is vital to strengthening love. Discovering one another's gifts, exploring new mutual interests, and investing together in other people's lives make marriage after 50 fabulous.

Opportunities abound for discovering new interests in marriage, whether enrolling in courses through a local college, taking up a companionable sport like hiking, signing up for trips or classes through Elderhostel, Inc., or working together on short-term mission projects. Finding a focus outside of oneself, learning to treasure the beauties of one's spouse, and investing together in others' lives will create new, stronger bonds in marriage. Making the marriage relationship a priority is vital for after-50 couples.

Being open with our husbands about bodily changes during menopause (see chapter 9)—hormonal issues, decreased sexual desire (perhaps due to painful intercourse), fluctuating body weight, and poor self-image—is crucial as we age. Being aware of our own feelings and also sharing them openly becomes necessary if we are to grow closer to our husbands during the second half of life. Nurturing one another and setting aside time to truly listen and dream together will help make marriage magnificent after 50.

Even so, the statistics show that "36 percent of women over age 65 live alone, and 24 percent of all U.S. households are made of single livers."[4] The divorce rate for 50-year-old women is 24 percent, and 43 percent of the total population of older Americans is single.[5] Since research shows that women tend to outlive men by ten years, there is a good possibility that most midlife women will be single at some point in the future. It's all the more crucial, then, to develop positive and powerful relationships with our children, grandchildren, and friends, and to find mentoring opportunities.

Your Children

Parenting has always been one of my most important and most rewarding roles. One year, on the Saturday before Mother's Day, I glanced out my window and saw a florist employee walking up my front walkway holding a stately bouquet of gorgeous yellow roses. I knew instantly that they were from my son David. Emotions welled up within me as the sight of those flowers transported me to another time.

When David had been a student at Auburn University, he had sent me a dozen exquisite yellow roses for Valentine's Day. Knowing his shoestring student budget, my eyes had filled with tears, and my heart with love, because of the love and care his thoughtfulness proved. I felt the strong arms of my champion wrestler son wrapping around me with warm compassion.

Several years later, when David married his radiant bride, Angela, I remembered his gift of unselfish love and filled the room for the rehearsal dinner with dozens of brilliant roses of every shade and hue. As David stepped into the elaborate room filled with love and roses, his eyes met mine, and I knew he understood my desire to give my pledge of love to him and his bride. The flickering glow of candlelight and the sweet fragrance of roses whispered through the room like a soft mist, giving the soon-to-be-newlyweds a golden glimpse of their future together.

In recent years, we have enjoyed three christening parties for David and Angela's precious children. The day after each baby's christening, I received yellow roses with a card that read, "Dear Grandmother Shirley, Thank you for making my christening party so special." Each had been "signed" Stephanie, Sarah, or Jackson.

That Saturday, as I opened the door to receive the flowers, I thought with a tearful smile, *Love never ends.* Burying my face in the baby-soft petals, I thought I heard a soft whisper, "I love you, Mother."

Though my nest is usually empty now, not every woman has an empty nest when she turns 50. With countless options available to women in their 20s, many wait to marry and have children until careers are established, homes purchased, and degrees finished. This means that many fabulous, 50-plus women will be attending PTA meetings and cheering at their ten-year-old's soccer games, all the while trying to deal with hormones and menopause and the host of other exciting but complicating midlife matters.

Other empty nests are not alone for long, with baby boomers having "boomerang" children—off to school, to work, and then back home again for a variety of reasons. Or perhaps the children are grown, with established households and careers, and the mother left alone feels neglected.

This is where our supportive network of friends and other vital, life-giving relationships and activities come into play. Rather than sit and wonder why the children don't call or visit, we build up our lives with meaningful relationships, visit our children when we can, and, as they say, "Get a life." Finding our focus after 50 frees up our children to live their own lives (even if we think they're running them badly!) and takes the burden off of them to be our sole sources of interest, meaning, love, and affirmation.

Your Grandchildren

Solomon, who presumably had many grandchildren, said, "*Grandchildren are the crown of old men*" (Proverbs 17:6). Perhaps this is because, with grandchildren, we get the chance to bask in the wonders of life all over again. "To show a child what once delighted you, to find the child's delight added to your own—this is happiness," said J. B. Priestley.

Finding enchantment in their precious minds and in their courageous, creative spirits increases our own quality of living, as well. One weekend, I had the joy of watching three of my grandchildren while my son David and his wife, Angela, took a much-needed mini-vacation. A loud, windy thunderstorm interrupted our dawn-till-dusk play. Seven-year-old Sarah, with two beautiful dimples in her gorgeous face, looked at me with frightened eyes.

Then, with a toss of her head, she said, "Lightning is angels playing with lightbulbs." Gathering courage from her own words, she went on, "Thunder is angels going bowling, and rain is God taking a bath, or God watering His flowers." I thanked God for the privilege of being a part of her life, even as those sweet dimples flashed out from behind her fear.

Grandparenting is a privilege and an enormous opportunity to share our wisdom and faith. James Dobson, Ph.D., founder of Focus on the Family, speaks of the faith of his grandmother and how it ultimately led him into a relationship with the Lord. A grandparent's faith is vital in bringing up future generations! In fact, Moses halted the Israelites at the edge of the Promised Land and repeated God's commandment:

> *Now this is the commandment, the statues and the judgments which the LORD your God has commanded me to teach you, that you might do them in the land where you are going over to possess it, so that you and your son and your grandson might fear the LORD your God, to keep all His statutes and His commandments, which I command you, all the days of your life, and that your days may be prolonged.* (Deuteronomy 6:1–2)

Not only do our grandchildren gain from being in relationship with us, but others gain, as well, from their childlike light, brightness, and joy. Corrie ten Boom aptly expressed the mutual benefits: "Children need the wisdom of their elders; the aging need the encouragement of a child's exuberance."[6]

Norma started taking a friend's son, Josh, on visits to the nursing home when he was just three. The residents responded with alertness and huge smiles, fondly reaching out to pat his head as he visited with each of them. Norma glowed with the chance to share her "grandson" with a group of people old enough to be Josh's great-grandparents, and Josh returned to his own family full of intergenerational stories and a more well-rounded understanding of aging and "extended family" in America. The U.S. Census Bureau reports that 3.7 million grandparents have brought their grandchildren into their own homes to raise; an additional one million grandparents have moved into their children's homes and are helping raise the grandchildren there. The number of grandchildren under the age of 18 who are living with grandparents has jumped 59 percent since 1980, to 3.9 million. Almost two-thirds of the grandparents living with their grandchildren are women.[7] What an opportunity to *"train up a child in the way he should go"* (Proverbs 22:6).

However, it can also be exhausting, draining, and disappointing to find oneself tasked with raising yet another generation of children. Elaine, for instance, dreamed of traveling after retirement from a teaching career, only to find herself providing daycare for all of her grandchildren. If you find yourself in a caregiving role, it is crucial that you have a support network in place, get further training, if necessary, to deal with special problems in parenting grandchildren, and recognize and care for your own needs.[8]

Parenting Your Parents

The slow drip of the IV nourished and medicated my father as he lay, seemingly lifeless, on the sterile, white hospital bed. Like a crown of glory, his white hair blended in with the white pillow. Staring at the frail form on the bed, I couldn't believe that, in his prime, my dad had weighed 200 pounds. I watched from a chair in the corner of the dimly lit room and remembered his younger, stronger body. My dad had always had excellent posture. He'd walked with an aura of confidence until a stroke had slowed his pace.

The dim, bleak mood of the hospital room changed with a mental flashback to Dad sweeping me off the ground in his hard, strong arms and whirling me around him when I was ten to prancing around a wagon pulled by a tractor and bearing a prized possession—my piano—and giggling, happily. Moving my piano from my grandparents' home next door to our new home, a house my dad had built with his own sweat and labor, was a thrill. As cotton farmers, my parents had to make every penny count. That fact that I could own a piano and take lessons was a miracle that could have happened only by divine providence, brought to life by parents who had dreamed and planned to make it happen. The highlight of my week came each Saturday morning when I walked two miles to my piano lesson. But the morning we moved my precious piano to our new home trumped even piano lessons in importance.

My dad, driving the tractor that pulled the wagon, failed to see the root of an old oak tree sticking up a few inches above the ground. The wagon hit the root with one wheel, dislodging the massive upright piano. It bounced out onto the hard ground and rolled over and over, breaking into a thousand splinters.

The magnitude of my loss sank deep into my soul. I started to run, screaming and crying. My dad caught me, picked me up in his strong arms, and hugged me to him as I beat upon his broad shoulders with my small, clenched fists. "You broke my piano!" I screamed in his ear.

He held my trembling body firmly to his bosom until I stopped sobbing. His big, green eyes looked deeply into my bewildered, dark brown ones. His face was sad, but he said, "Before I die, I will buy you a new piano."

A decade went by, and then another. I moved into a new home with my husband and three children. One day, the doorbell rang. A piano salesman introduced himself. "Your dad has paid for any piano you would like," he said, handing me a catalog filled with all kinds of pianos. Through my tears, I selected my favorite.

I love playing my piano. My children learned to play on it, and now my grandchildren press the ivory keys. That piano occupies a special place, in my living room and in my heart. This special place in my heart is also filled with sadness because I miss my dad, whose home is now in heaven.

Increasingly, baby boomers may find themselves part of the so-called "sandwich generation." With older people living longer and healthier lives, many of our parents are still alive when we turn 50. It is likely that we will become the caregivers of our own parents. Statistics from the U.S. Census Bureau point out that nearly one million adults live with their adult children, with grandchildren in the home, as well.[9]

Many parents are relieved when grandparents come in and help with the raising of the children, shuttling, errands, and housework. But it also brings increasing complexity and confusion, as personalities, needs, and values may differ among the various adults in the home. Since the health of the grandparents who move in with the parents and grandkids may be poorer, this often compromises one's energy level and the use of one's time, as well. Once again, in the midst of demanding relationships, it is vital to stay in close contact with our own needs and feelings, maintain supportive friendships, and keep close to God for wisdom and strength. Honoring our parents as we raise our own children is important.

Your Friendships

Midlife is a good time to examine our friendships. If we find ourselves constantly on the listening end, we may ask ourselves if the other person is truly a friend. A friend really listens to us and doesn't feel compelled to immediately jump in and reclaim control of the conversation with, "I know what you mean. Just the other day...." Friends are not threatened by our success—or by our failure. Friends are there for the work and for the fun. Friends pick us up when we are down for the count; if we're too heavy, they get down alongside us.

A real friend affirms us. Even though a senior may have high self-esteem, everyone looks for and profits from affirmation. Friends energize us. Friends ask us hard questions and love us even when we don't get the answers right. They listen thoroughly, challenge us to live out our dreams and use our gifts, and encourage us to grow. Carolyn has done this for me. We have laughed till our sides ached, cried on each other's shoulders, worked together, played together, and created memories that will last a lifetime.

One of the best ways to grow is to seek out friends who are role models for us—people who challenge us to grow *better* as we grow older. Friends can also be for us what we may not have in our transient society—family. It's not too late to find a surrogate sister, or six of them.

The movie *Steel Magnolias* grips the viewer with its theme of friendship. Olympia Dukakis, one of the costars, describes "the cement bond of friendship" as a group of women moving together through life's ups and downs, surrounding one another with support, love, and humor.

We each have a longing for a deeper connection. Our great, relational God, three-in-one, created us for relationships—with family, with friends, and with Himself. He also created us to be mentors and role models for others.

Your Mentors

George Bernard Shaw said, "I want to be thoroughly used up when I die, for the harder I work, the more I live. Life is no brief candle for me. It is a splendid torch which I have got hold of for the moment, and I want to make it burn as brightly as possible before handing it on to future generations."

Carol decided that, in order to hand off the torch to future generations, she needed to resign from high-profile, "do everything" volunteer work and train other people to take her place. She then began to invest deeply in one life at a time. This fabulous, 50-plus woman abandoned the excuse "But I need more training," realizing God had placed her for years in one-on-one relationships. The high-profile work began to seem empty and wearying as she developed deeper connections with younger women.

Carol also set up a program in her church called the Venus Project, named after a young woman whose life was snuffed out too soon. The Venus Project paired up women from different generations, with the goal of enabling the older women to guide the younger ones.

Business professionals figured this out long ago. Take an expert who's been working successfully in the field for years and put him in the classroom at the graduate level to teach from experience. For Mary, her life experiences also took her back to school; every week, she volunteers in the local high school cafeteria. "I miss my grandchildren," she says. "This way, I can give back to the youth, build into their lives, pay attention, and just love them. I think it makes a difference. It certainly makes a difference in my life!"

Whether we pass the torch through one-on-one mentoring or broader work with a group, "It's all about the other person," says Claudia, who works for a major social service agency in the large gifts department. "When I talk with someone about a contribution, it's not about how much money I can convince him or her to donate. It's learning about the other's interests and passions, and helping figure out a perfect fit. I love it!" She sees her work as a ministry—a means of passing on to others that life-giving torch.

• LIMITLESS LIVING •

Enormous joy and satisfaction are possible for the 50-plus woman who chooses to invest in others. Regardless of past pain and the potential for future problems, giving our love and energy to others expands the boundaries of our lives. When we choose to love, in spite of risk, we win the aging game.

• QUESTIONS FOR IMMEDIATE APPLICATION •

1. List three ways you will become more comfortable in your own skin and appreciate the wonderful woman you have turned out to be.
2. List three creative ways you will enjoy your relationships more, starting with your family—specifically, your children and grandchildren.
3. How will you invest your time and attention in your long-time friends while also making new ones?

• TOP TEN FAVORITE RELATIONSHIP STRATEGIES •

1. Make time for your friends. They will extend and expand your life.
2. Nothing feels better than having someone interested in you. Ask questions to learn all you can about another person's interests, gifts, roles, needs, and dreams.
3. Practice setting boundaries. For instance, how often do you cancel your plans at the last minute in order to babysit the grandchildren at the last minute?
4. Figure out your own needs and expectations in relationships.
5. Work on self-awareness so that you may then be "other-aware."
6. List the roles you fill and the relationships you have. Where are the gaps?

7. We find happiness when we serve. Where are you giving to others?
8. Pay attention to your conversations with others. Who does most of the talking? Why?
9. Prioritize your relationships from most important and life-giving to the least.
10. Don't expect others to make you feel good about yourself. That comes only from knowing you are precious and beloved in God's eyes!

AGING SUCCESSFULLY: ATTITUDE #6

Investing in relationships for eternity gives our lives depth, breadth, and a reason for living well.

CHAPTER 7

DEBUNKING THE DIET MYSTERIES: EATING RIGHT

"My sense of wonder at the beauty of our body's ability to take the foodstuffs from our dining room tables and shape them to our complex purposes is profound. A grape helps me frame a new idea. Amazing! A lamb chop fuels the morning jog. Wonderful! A glass of milk becomes part of my femur. Terrific!"

—Walter M. Bortz II, M.D.[1]

"A merry heart hath a continual feast."

—Proverbs 15:15 (KJV)

Aging means constant change, like shifting shadows on a windy, moonlit night. The shades of change can be exciting, magic, and fruitful if we focus on the positive facets. Age may become a dance of mounting intrigue and new horizons.

Malcom Gillis of Toney, Alabama, held the world record in 1994 for his age group in the half marathon (13.1 miles). At 60, he has three secrets to successful aging:

1. Stay extremely active and have many interests in life.
2. Eat sparingly to stay thin.
3. Eat little or no meat. (Mr. Gillis is a vegetarian.)

This champion runner participates in marathons all over the world. Each day offers a fresh chance to push out of the starting blocks, and he enjoys every day of his age.

Like Mr. Gillis, people who embrace change with a positive attitude, proper diet, and daily exercise will make the "fab 50s" a prime time of life. Becoming a willing partner in the dance of change requires saying no to wallflower behavior. Life will sideline us if we passively accept the negative stereotypes of aging.

All this dancing, however, takes energy, a priceless commodity for the young as well as the young at heart. Energy is the power surge that keeps us young and active. Four basic practices will keep our energy high:

1. A *balanced diet* undergirds good health, which is the trump card of aging and energy.
2. *Exercise* is the golden egg of aging and energy (the subject of the next chapter).
3. *Enthusiasm* enhances aging.
4. *Staying in control of our life*, beginning by recognizing Jesus Christ as our captain. This allows us to lead independent, energetic lives. Energy squeals, "I'm excited to be alive! I'm excited about life!"

Just before addressing a meeting, I felt about as exciting to the audience as a bowl of overcooked oatmeal. I went into the ladies' room and visualized the enthusiastic speaker who could motivate and encourage any audience. I jumped up and down to kick-start my energy. I thought rhapsodic, positive thoughts, and put an eager look on my face. My speech was full of fire, and my audience loved it.

If your energy level always seems low, examine your lifestyle. Center your life around things you enjoy, pursue challenging goals, and spend time with people you care about. Keep active. Say yes to new experiences. Stretch yourself to serve others and enjoy every precious minute of this extraordinary life.

• AVOID ENERGY ZAPPERS •

Some of the biggest energy zappers include lack of exercise, lack of sleep, and lack of the ability to maintain a vision. Furthermore, boredom, poor health, stress, imbalanced diet, dormant faith, and having nothing to look forward to are also energy zappers. Skipping breakfast, another zapper, is something women across America tend to do, for weight control as well as for time management. Skipping this all-important meal actually slows our metabolism and causes undue strain on the digestive process when we finally eat a meal later in the day. A good breakfast is the spark that gets the fire going in our metabolism.

To boost our overall health, we should avoid these energy zappers. Nutrition, exercise, discipline, time, and hard work are part of the formula for fitness after 50. Setting attainable goals for improved fitness, planning, and then working the plan will push us toward personal excellence.

In planning for fitness, three areas must be recognized: diet, exercise, and mental attitude. Basic knowledge of nutrition and exercise, combined with a positive mental attitude, are essentials in any fitness program. Planning for fitness, today's older women have everything to gain and nothing to lose—except some extra baggage. Nothing weighs us down more than a heavy spirit, and moving our metabolism up a notch through improved nutrition and fitness will lift our spirits and lighten the physical load we carry, as well.

A positive, day-to-day approach to healthful living produces optimal physical and mental well-being. There is no magic method to living longer, says Dr. Robert Belihar of the National Wellness and Longevity Center in Davidson County, Tennessee.[2] "It has to do with fitness, nutrition, and to a certain extent, medication. We can make ourselves younger by the foods we eat."

• HOW MUCH IS ENOUGH? •

The concept of getting younger by eating right is good news, assuming we eat! In a time of increasing anorexia among aging women,[3] it's important to address the issue of weight. Women, unfortunately, are too often obsessed with weight, whether it's an extra five pounds now and then or true obesity. You have lived in your body for years. You know it like no one else. You can look in the mirror, honestly, and tell if you have been eating too much or unwisely. Your body tells you when you are hungry and low on energy. Listen to your body.

Walter M. Bortz II, M.D., says, "...the old machine needs pretty much the same amount and type of food that the younger machine does, providing it is well maintained and fit."[4] Many doctors recommend that we make our weight at age 18 our target weight, assuming that it works with our bone structure and height.

True obesity is obvious to everyone. It adds years to our age, slows us down, and is linked with hypertension, arthritis, elevated cholesterol, and diabetes. Obesity also gives women of any age a battle with self-image. We must eat smart!

• FABULOUS WOMEN EAT SMART •

The remainder of this chapter was written with Debra K. Goodwin, R.D., L.D., a registered dietitian who teaches nutrition at Jacksonville State University, Jacksonville, Alabama.

Paramount to fitness is a balanced diet. Many women live as if eating were abnormal. Our society's emphasis on extreme thinness has forced some individuals to severely curtail their intake of valuable nutrients, which may disastrously affect their health and definitely influences their vitality.

Building a fit body begins on the inside. A self-assured look isn't all attitude. A woman stands tall only as a natural response from strong bones.

Avoiding Osteoporosis

One battle the 50-and-beyond woman fights is against osteoporosis, a condition in which the bones begin to lose density and become weak, vulnerable to breakage. Unfortunately, because osteoporosis is a silent disease, a woman's first warning may come when she steps off a curb—and breaks a hip. Although heredity may increase the likelihood of some aging women to have osteoporosis, there are ways to fight this disease.

The hormone estrogen aids in building women's bones by locking calcium inside them. Hormone replacement therapy remains a valid option for rebuilding bone density and stopping osteoporosis. In addition, extra calcium intake throughout life is vital for building strong bones and teeth.

Milk mustaches became chic in 1995, when the National Fluid Milk Processor Promotion Board launched a new ad campaign to educate women on the number one nutritional problem in America. Celebrities such as Lauren Bacall, Christie Brinkley, and even Mark Maguire sported the white foam in magazine ads. David McCarron, a professor of medicine at Oregon Health Sciences University, says that 75 percent of women do not get the minimum daily requirement of calcium. Unfortunately, this includes even weight-conscious teenagers, many of whom opt for a one-calorie diet drink instead of milk as their beverage of choice. They are laying a weak foundation for their future.

If you are fighting the bulge, you may choose to get your calcium from a skinny glass of skim milk. Smart drinking means replacing soft drinks, coffee, and nonnutritious drinks and their empty calories with milk and water. "You've certainly lost weight," I remarked to a dear lady named Sharon I'd seen at the supermarket. "How did you do it?"

Her sheepish grin delighted me. "I quit drinking colas. That's it. I substituted water for pop and lost 35 pounds." She looked like a new woman, and she exuded a renewed sense of energy, purpose, and confidence.

Along with calcium, foods rich in boron are vital. "Research at the USDA Grand Forks Human Nutrition Research Center in North Dakota shows that boron may slow bone loss in the critical years following menopause. Good sources of boron include apples, nuts, raisins, legumes, grape juice, and green vegetables."[5] According to Dr. Christiane Northrup, boron may reduce urinary calcium loss and increase serum levels of 17-beta estradiol; both effects help bone health. The 2 mg. per day MDR is easily met through diet.[6]

An active lifestyle and daily exercise also strengthen bones. "French researchers have shown that 35 weeks in bed provoke the same amount of calcium loss from the bones as seen in ten years of aging."[7]

Other Important Ingredients in a Good Diet

In general, today's maturing woman should pay close attention not only to calcium and boron but also to iron, fiber, folate, and vitamin E.

Iron is important for oxygen transportation in the body and thus the release of energy. "Iron-poor blood" causes fatigue. Eat lean meats, dried fruits, and whole grain breads. Watch, however, megadoses of iron, as too much iron has an aging effect. Most Americans consume more than adequate amounts of iron through fortified cereals and other foods; additional iron is rarely recommended unless prescribed by a doctor.

Fiber, another vital ingredient, decreases the risk of colon cancer and heart disease. It also helps to maintain the health and tone of the digestive tract. Twenty-five to 35 grams of fiber per day are recommended. Whole grain breads, many of fruits and vegetables, dried beans, and peas contain high levels of fiber.

Two other nutrients that may contribute to preventing heart disease, which is a threat for the post-menopausal woman, are folate and vitamin E. Research suggests that these two nutrients may need to be supplemented in the diet.

The immune system is definitely eavesdropping on what's going on in your life. You have to be healthy to look your best, so it's important to eat a balanced diet. Glowing, silky hair and clear skin are by-products of a nutritious diet. Although no specific food will prevent wrinkles from forming on your face, maintaining a healthy weight and eating a balanced diet will ease facial lines and make your skin glow.

Follow the Food Plate

In 2012, the USDA replaced the traditional food pyramid with the new food plate. The food plate is a visual representation of the daily foods that individuals should eat for good health. Three fourths of the plate should consist in plant-based foods, such as fruits, vegetables, and grain products (such as bread, pasta, and cereals). The remaining fourth of the plate contains low-fat proteins, such as meat, poultry, fish, and dried beans or peas. Dairy products, such as milk, cheese, and yogurt, are represented by a smaller plate on the side. The emphasis of the new food plate is a balanced diet through consumption of more plant-based foods and smaller portions.

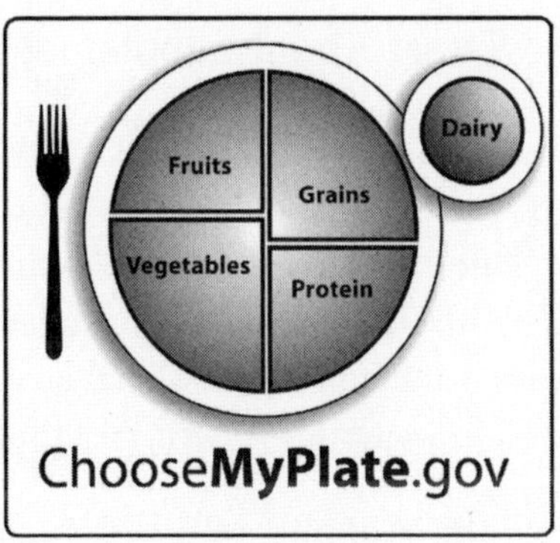

Fresh, natural, unprocessed foods are key in a nutritious diet. Preparation methods such as steaming, baking, and broiling conserve nutrients and fiber, keep calories low, and enhance the flavor of foods.

The food plate reminds us to limit our intake of both fat and sodium. In general, the more highly processed the food, the higher the fat and sodium contents. If in doubt, read the labels and packaging. The American Heart Association recommends that less than 30 percent of our daily calories be derived from fat.[8] We need this much fat, however, to cushion and protect our vital organs, maintain hormonal balance, give our skin and hair a healthy glow, support cell walls, provide energy, and circulate the fat-soluble vitamins A, D, E, and K.

Eating for optimal health means eating smart snacks for quick energy pickups, and therefore eating more frequently throughout the day. Pamela M. Smith, R.D., suggests eating "fresh fruit, raisins, low-fat cheese or yogurt, a half sandwich, or even a trail mix of dry-roasted peanuts and sunflower seeds mixed with dried fruit." These power snacks prevent ravenous hunger (we make poorer food choices in the throes of a craving or hunger spell) and keep our blood sugar at a normal level.[9]

Be Smart About Supplements

Michael Roizen, author of *RealAge*, recommends supplementing our daily diet with only five vitamins and minerals: calcium (1000-1200mg), vitamins C (600mg or more, plus two servings through diet), D (400IU), E (400IU), and folate (400 mcg). (C, D, E, and folate: just remember the alphabet, he says).[10] Roizen also recommends a low-vitamin A, iron-free multivitamin daily.

Be Wary of Fad Diets

Special diets generate a great deal of hype and interest among people seeking to lose weight fast. One of these diets, a high-protein, high-fat, low- to zero-carbohydrate plan, assures its followers of rapid weight loss and a return of energy.

What we may not realize, however, is that a high-protein (meat-based) diet, unless counterbalanced with dairy products, may leech calcium from bones. In addition, it stresses the kidneys, whose job it is to excrete extra protein. Since the body will utilize only the protein it needs, much of the excess is shipped off to the kidneys, which work overtime to get rid of it. (Some protein turns into fat and sugars in the body.)[11]

In general, a fad diet makes absurd promises. Avoid focusing on any specific food or food group and eschew any diet that forces you to buy a specialty food product. The "next-day" miracle diet is a miracle only for the person pocketing the money from sales. Remember, if it sounds too good to be true, it probably is!

Water, Water Everywhere

Our bodies, properly hydrated, should be 74 percent water,[13] and water is the basis of all body fluids: digestive juices, blood, urine, lymph, and perspiration. Cell processes and organ functions depend on water. It is essential for lubrication and is the basis for saliva and mucous secretions. Water bathes the joints, keeps food moving through the intestinal tract to eliminate waste and prevent constipation, and helps regulate body temperature. In addition, water deprivation is linked to fatigue and to slow mind/thought processes, because the majority of the human brain is water. Water is an easy energy booster!

In fact, Dr. Gary Null treats patients with dementia first by giving them large amounts of cold water throughout the day for three weeks. After that time, he begins to see their dementia dissipate because they've rehydrated their brains. Water increases neuron activity and better cellular chemistry at any age.[14]

We may live several weeks without food, but we can survive only a few days without water.

To keep your fluids well balanced, drink six to eight (8-ounce) glasses of water. Plain old tap water will do, although both city and well water should be checked to ensure they contain healthy levels of trace elements. Juice, milk, and soup can provide some of your daily water needs; however, coffee, tea, and soda are not good substitutes for water because of their diuretic effect.

Adequate water intake helps keep hands, feet, and legs from swelling. When we're stingy with our water consumption, our body notices, and it then stores every extra drop outside the cells, thus causing water retention, or bloating.

Keeping our bodies hydrated helps maintain muscle tone and plumps our skin, making it healthy and resilient. Keeping a glass of water near your primary work area may help remind you to stay hydrated. Lynn, when dusting one afternoon, noticed her crystal stemware sparkling in the sun. Remembering her doctor's admonition to drink more water, she filled a water goblet and brought it to her desk in her home office so she could sip in style. She claims that the extra water helps her thinking, her energy, and even her sex life!

• SPIRITUAL FITNESS •

To become totally fit, the aging person will find that living water enhances every aspect of life. In other words, our spiritual fitness is just as important as our physical fitness, if not more so. While sitting at Jacob's well one day, Jesus asked a Samaritan woman for a drink of water. She said, *"How can you ask me for a drink?"* (John 4:9 NIV). She knew that social and religious laws of the time prohibited men from speaking with women, especially women with her moral track record.

> *Jesus answered her, "If you knew the gift of God and who it is that asks you for a drink, you would have asked him and he would have given you living water."* (John 4:10 NIV)

Jesus went on to say, *"Whoever drinks of the water I give him will never thirst. Indeed, the water I give him will become...a spring of water welling up to eternal life"* (John 4:14 NIV).

Along with our physical food, God gives us spiritual food. Jesus said, *"I am the bread of life;* [s]*he who comes Me shall not hunger and* [s]*he who believes in Me shall never thirst"* (John 6:35). Even in paradise, He will feed us. *"To him* [her] *who overcomes, I will grant to eat of the tree of life, which is in Paradise of God"* (Revelation 2:7).

And the water analogy continues, even to eternity:

> *And the* LORD *shall guide thee continually, and satisfy thy soul in drought, and make fat thy bones: and thou shalt be like a watered garden, and like a spring of water, whose waters fail not.* (Isaiah 58:11 KJV)

That seems to be the success formula of ageless living: tapping into the Source of living water, which keeps us healthy from here to eternity.

• QUESTIONS FOR IMMEDIATE APPLICATION •

1. How do you feel about your current diet? What would you like to change? If you struggle with overeating or undereating, try keeping a food journal, in which you record your emotions and what you eat, in order to search for patterns in the relationship between the way you feel and the way you eat in response.
2. What has been your experience with various types of diets and weight-loss methods?
3. If you could change one thing about your eating habits, what would it be? How would you do it?

• TOP TEN STRATEGIES FOR EATING RIGHT •

1. Be realistic. Don't try to revamp your entire dietary lifestyle in a single week.
2. Start with something simple: drink lots of water.
3. Moderation is key in most things. Eating is no exception. Practice moderation!
4. Special diets that focus on a particular food group or type of food do not promote balance in eating.

5. Remember, if it sounds too good to be true ("Lose 50 pounds by Tuesday! Guaranteed!"), it probably is.
6. Limit, don't eliminate. Don't cut out foods you love; just limit your consumption of them.
7. Eat more small meals throughout the day to keep your energy level more stable.
8. Don't skip breakfast!
9. Remember, the fresher the food, the closer it is to its original form and the better it is for you.
10. Don't deprive yourself. Remember that eating is normal behavior. If you are eating for emotional comfort or from stress, try journaling to get a handle on what's eating you!

AGING SUCCESSFULLY: ATTITUDE #7

Excellent nutrition energizes me to live agelessly.

CHAPTER 8

FITNESS AFTER 50

"If we don't use our muscles, hearts, and brains, they'll shrivel."

–Dr. Walter Bortz II

"Moses was 120 years old when he died, yet his eyesight was perfect and he was as strong as a young man."

–Deuteronomy 34:7 (TLB)

Vim and vigor at 50 puts you on pitch to sing the song of successful aging, and zip requires a fit body. A fit body can't be bought, but the good news is, women in middle life can build muscle, gain strength, and increase their stamina and flexibility. We can discard one of the common myths of aging: atrophy and crippling are *not* inevitable.

With the proper exercise plan, our generation can retard or repel the ravages of disease, aging, and gravity. Fitness for older women is imperative, if we are to believe current T-shirt wisdom: "If you don't take care of your body, where will you live?" All of the goal-oriented information in the rest of this book is worthless if our bodies are not fit enough to carry out our dreams.

Exercise, combined with sound nutrition and an upbeat attitude, offers an unbeatable formula for vigor in midlife. After perusing recent research and realizing how great are the benefits of exercise on health, attitude, and longevity, I feel it is safe to say, "Exercise or die."

Unfortunately, not many of us take up the challenge to improve our physical well-being. Data from the Centers for Disease Control shows only 16 percent of women 65 or older exercised regularly in 1990, and this percentage decreases as women age. Mike Snider wrote in *USA Today*, "If the USA got a grade for exercise, it probably would be 'd' for darned little."[1]

In the age of "instant"—instant oatmeal, instant cash, instant telecommunication—many find it frustrating to develop a long-term plan for fitness. Instant fitness is not possible, but the rewards of consistent workouts are tremendous.

• WORKOUT REWARDS •

1. *Increased Energy*: Exercise strengthens the lungs, dilates blood vessels, pushes toxins out of our bodies through sweat, mobilizes energy stores, and allows blood to flow more freely.
2. *Cardiovascular Conditioning*: Exercise strengthens the heart. A fit heart transports oxygen with greater efficiency to all parts of the body, providing more stamina as it maximizes nutrient supply. Because postmenopausal women are at a greater risk for heart disease, you should consult your physician about taking an aspirin daily to further benefit the heart. This simple practice may cut the risk of heart attack in half.
3. *Increased Metabolism*: Exercise burns fat faster, partly because it increases metabolism, and partly because it builds muscle, which burns calories at a faster rate than fat does.
4. *Increased Brain Function*: Dr. Walter M. Bortz II, former president of the Geriatrics Society, believes exercise improves blood circulation to the brain and stimulates the formation

and release of noradrenaline. Brain stimulation results when the brain is bathed with higher levels of noradrenaline.

5. *Decreased Stress:* The worry-hurry habit leads to stress, and stress is the road to pain, as well as a leading contributor to America's number one killer: heart disease. Symptoms of stress include feelings of panic, a knotted stomach, headaches, a pounding heart, the inability to concentrate, nervous gestures, and insomnia, as well as the perception that life is out of control. Exercise is an effective stress-buster, reenergizing the body and acting as a safety valve for our roiling internal anxieties.

   Jesus is also an excellent "stress-buster." He said, "*Come unto me, all ye that labour and are heavy laden, and I will give you rest. Take my yoke upon you, and learn of me; for I am meek and lowly in heart: and ye shall find rest unto your souls. For my yoke is easy, and my burden is light*" (Matthew 11:28–30 KJV).

6. *Fluidity of Movement:* Elastic isn't just for the pants of middle-aged people! As we age, our muscles lose their elasticity. Gentle stretching helps us regain our flexibility and keeps us supple. It also alleviates stiffness and rigidity, which, in turn, reduces the risk of injury from moving or lifting.

   As Dr. Bortz concisely summarizes, the benefits of exercise affect:

   > ...body weight, blood pressure, HDL cholesterol (the beneficial kind), blood clotting, respiratory function, heart muscle strength, muscle mass, bone density, obesity, intestinal function, sexual capacity, glucose tolerance, immunologic capacity, and behavioral characteristics such as mood, cognition, and memory.[2]

With all these benefits in mind, let's explore the array of options available to us as we determine to be fit after 50.

• OPTIONS FOR EXERCISE •

The market is flooded with possibilities for fitness.

Workouts on DVDs

Perhaps the simplest mode of exercise for the unmotivated or those who don't know where to begin is a workout on DVD. These resources help us through our shyness in the beginning stages of exercise, when we're tempted to say, "I'm too uncoordinated/out of shape/overweight/etc. to work out with real people." These DVDs provide safe workouts in a nonthreatening environment (our homes). An added benefit is that the fashion police won't come to call, and so we need not worry about our stretched-out sweats and sloppy shirts, nor must we replace them with the latest Spandex.

Judi Sheppard Missett has helped many women get fit and stay fit. As president of Jazzercise, Inc., she has transformed workout routines into energetic, fun, motivating, upbeat, mood-changing, total-body conditioning through her dance DVDs. These routines put a smile on your face and excitement in your stride, no matter your age. Judi's exercise DVDs live out her philosophy that exercise should be both fun and effective.

Most libraries have shelves of exercise DVDs, making it easy to try various workouts, from low-impact to high-impact aerobics to stretching, toning, and spot exercising (such as Greg Smithey's *Buns of Steel*). In addition, some television channels feature daily workouts with a physical trainer.

Group Workouts

For the people person, as well as the person needing accountability, group workouts are an excellent choice. Check the availability of exercise classes senior citizen centers and athletic clubs. Your local YMCA probably offers many levels and types of exercise classes. Hospitals are also leaping on the exercise wagon, opening fitness centers with specialized programs for midlifers. Many community centers have new groups aimed at the baby boomers, that ever-burgeoning market of people who want to feel and look better so they may keep moving and keep changing the world! The group setting also functions as a place for socialization, thus decreasing the isolation and resulting depression aging often brings.

Sessions with a Personal Trainer

Formerly considered an option for the rich and famous alone, a personal trainer is now available in most local gyms and fitness centers to help develop a personalized routine for each individual and to work through that routine with the client regularly. This individualized attention and accountability have helped me tremendously, keeping me exercising when I might otherwise have given up.

Dr. Bortz recommended that I work with a trainer so I could keep lifting my grandbabies, and it's been working! With three sessions a week, I feel tighter, stronger, and more energized, plus my clothes fit better! I use strength resistance equipment and end each workout on a cardiovascular machine, such as a treadmill or elliptical. I started on the cardio machine with three minutes of huffing and puffing. After a year, I was out breezing through 35 minutes of cardio! Thanks the sessions with my trainer, I'm getting younger by the day!

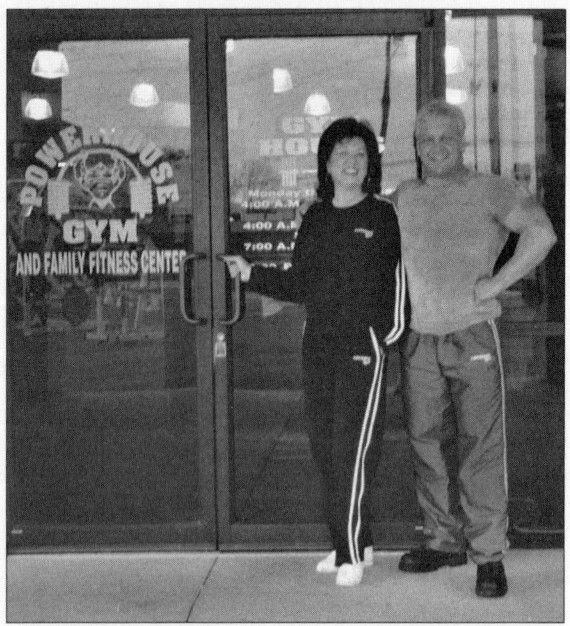

Shirley with trainer Eddie Underwood at the Power House Gym, where she works out

• FOUR FITNESS AREAS TO FOCUS ON •

Whether we exercise in a private or public setting, experts strongly recommend four areas of fitness on which to focus: stamina, strength, stretching, and balance. This combination results in a fit body able to withstand, or at least delay, the normal declines of aging.

> When aging promotes a gradual physical decline starting in middle age, a terrible downward spiral often ensues... feeling weak leads us to become more sedentary, and this inactivity in turn leads to further frailty. This spiral often leads to total dependence on others, loneliness, and isolation.[3]

Fortunately, severe physical decline is not inevitable, and it is reversible with a few minutes of attention to fitness each day. Michael Roizen, author of *RealAge*, claims that a 20-minute boost in physical activity every day, even if you don't break a sweat, reduces the risk of heart attack and stroke by 15 to 30 percent in just 20 weeks.[4]

Stamina

A 30-minute aerobic workout three times a week is ideal for cardiovascular conditioning. By age 75, women have a 15 to 20 percent lower aerobic capacity than men of the same age,[5] but again, in only a few minutes a day, we can all improve our stamina by elevating both our heart rate and our breathing. Elevating these rates so that we sweat for 20 minutes three times a week is a vital anti-ager.[6]

Moderate exercises that boost stamina include swimming, bicycling, stationary cycling, gardening, walking, golfing (without a cart), tennis (doubles), volleyball, rowing, dancing, and even mopping or scrubbing the floor. Once you're in better shape, for more vigorous endurance activities, consider climbing stairs or hills, shoveling snow, briskly biking up hills, digging holes, playing singles tennis, swimming laps, cross-country skiing, downhill skiing, hiking, or jogging.[7]

Walking is an activity we can begin at any age, regardless of our physical condition, and so I'd like to discuss that activity in greater detail.

Many doctors recommend walking at least 20 minutes a day. Walking is the easiest exercise program to begin. You can walk anywhere, anytime, without having to pay for a fitness club membership or purchase high-priced equipment. Committing to just 30 minutes a day, three days a week, assures us of adequate aerobic conditioning. Walking is also an insurance policy against a crumbling skeleton, as it minimizes and combats osteoporosis by actually strengthening our bones.

A healthy walk workout starts with good posture. Maintaining correct posture shaves years off of our appearance. Combining good posture with exercise brings us an appealing, years-younger look. For proper posture, stand erect, keep your chin parallel to the ground, and pull your head back so that your neck is in alignment with your spine. Pull your shoulder blades together and relax your shoulders and hips. One fashion expert says she imagines a hook pulling her up from the crown of her head, which aligns the rest of the body. Tuck in your tummy and straighten your spine, pulling your buns in so that the small of your back doesn't sway or bow. Expect to feel uncomfortable and awkward-looking for a while as you practice good posture. To test your posture, stand with your back against a wall and see how much of your back and shoulders touches the wall. Lifting your arms out to either side provides a stretch, as well as an additional posture checkpoint.

With the proper posture in place, begin your walking experience. Shoes designed for walking are a good investment. Beyond that, you should dress appropriately for the workout, expecting to shed a layer as you warm up. After gently limbering up, start moving!

Take quicker and shorter strides to jar the body less. Step with the heel leading. Bend your arms at 90-degree angles and allow them to swing naturally.

Dorothy, diagnosed at age 60 with dangerously high blood pressure, took a pricey prescription for her condition until her insurance no longer covered the cost. With her doctor's approval and monitoring, she bought a pair of good walking shoes and hit the road. Within one month of regular walking, Dorothy lowered her blood pressure and her cholesterol to a normal level, went off of the medication, improved her overall fitness, and brightened her outlook on life. Now a spry, energetic, healthy lady, she views her walk as the highlight of her day.

Strength

Weight lifting is not just for those who want a buff body at the beach. Though we lose one quarter to one third of a pound of muscle per year after age 35, according to Miriam Nelson, Ph.D., a scientist and specialist in aging at Tufts University, "Biologically we can reverse the aging process by 15 to 25 years."[10]

We do that by becoming stronger. Muscle-strengthening exercises are vital for the young, and the young at heart. According to the National Institute on Aging, "most people lose 20 to 40 percent of their muscle tissue as they get older."[11] Keeping our bodies strong helps ward off the general wear and tear of aging. Roizen suggests that even ten minutes of lifting weights, three times weekly, makes us 1.7 years younger.[12] Strength exercises fight off frailty and infirmity, keeping us independent. Strengthening exercises are especially crucial for women, helping protect bone mass and density.

Participants in one exercise study showed a 5 percent increase in strength with each exercise session.[13] One nursing home began a weight lifting program for its residents and soon had to close an entire wing of the facility because the participants had gotten stronger and gone home! The results of strength training are almost immediate, and they affect other areas of exercise, as well. Studies show that increasing our strength also increases our desire to incorporate other forms of exercise into our routine.

Major areas to focus on in strengthening exercises are the biceps, triceps, quadriceps, abdominals, hamstrings, and calf muscles.[14] Using some form of resistance, perform eight to 12 repetitions with a light weight to warm up your muscles for the first set. Build up to as many as three sets, increasing the weights used in each of the next two sets of repetitions. Perform each rep slowly, and resist the weight on the return to maximize the benefit.

Stretching

Our muscles begin to lose flexibility after age 40, if not sooner. The downhill slide can be redirected, however, decreasing the occurrence of common muscle strains, tears, and pulls. While stretching doesn't increase strength or endurance, it is vital for continued movement. Experts recommend stretching *after* the muscles have warmed up through strengthening or stamina-building exercises. Here are some stretching guidelines:

- If you have undergone a hip replacement, check with your doctor before performing any lower body stretching or exercises.
- Warm up before stretching to avoid injury.
- Stretching should be pain free; if you experience pain, ease up on the stretch until it no longer hurts. Mild discomfort or pulling is normal.
- No bouncing allowed! Perform slow, steady movements only; bouncing or jerking can cause muscle injury.
- Don't lock your joints into position but keep a tiny bend.[16]

Balance

A fourth key area for older adults to focus on in exercise is balance, the lack of which contributes to slips, falls, and breaks. Many strengthening (weight training) exercises also build balance.

Sarah, 58, stands on one foot and then the other for 20 seconds at a time, lightly touching a countertop for support. She also stands behind a chair and raises up on her tiptoes as high as possible, holding the pose for a few seconds, then lowers slowly. Her third balance exercise is walking heel-to-toe in a line, with heel and toe almost touching. Repeating these exercises eight to 15 times takes only minutes, but Sarah has found that devoting these minutes on a daily basis has increased her confidence dramatically.

Many senior centers and exercise facilities hold courses for older adults. Look into classes that would suit your physical needs.

• FEARFULLY AND WONDERFULLY MADE •

"Exercise," writes Michael Roizen, "is a whole-body phenomenon. It doesn't just make your muscles stronger; it slows down the aging of your entire body. Exercise affects everything: your cardiovascular system, your immune system, your musculoskeletal system, and your emotional well-being. It affects you all the way down to your cells."[18]

What a superb feeling to be alive in a healthy body! To take control of our health and well-being in only minutes a day seems either miraculous or ridiculous. But the studies don't lie. Exercise can rekindle our fire for life. What a remarkable return on our investment! With a healthy respect for our bodies, we can say with the psalmist, "*I am fearfully and wonderfully made...and my soul knows it very well*" (Psalm 139:14).

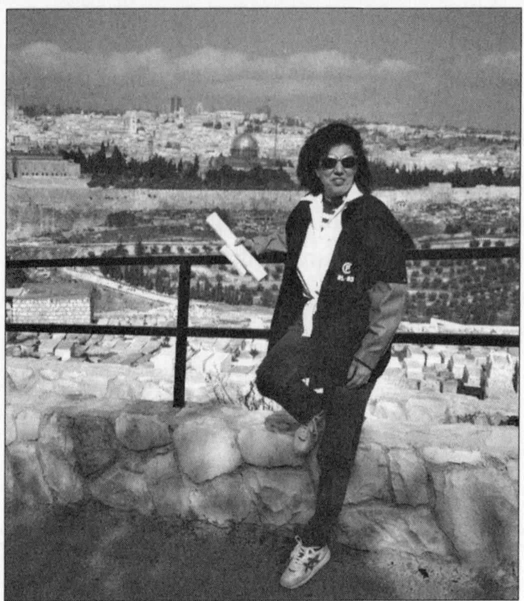

Shirley on a hike in the Holy Land

The National Institute on Aging offers a wide range of complimentary materials on aging well, including a booklet entitled "Exercise & Physical Activity: Your Everyday Guide form the National Institute on Aging." You may view this and other helpful booklets online at www.nia.nih.gov/health/pulication. You also have the option of ordering a print copy.

• QUESTIONS FOR IMMEDIATE APPLICATION •

1. What are you currently doing to improve your physical well-being? How do you feel about your level of fitness? In which of the four areas discussed are you the most fit—stretching, strength, stamina, or balance?
2. What is most appealing about beginning/improving an exercise plan? Most distasteful?

3. What motivations do you have, personally, to commit to better fitness? What goals can you set for yourself today? Who can help hold you accountable to a new plan?

• TOP TEN SHAPE-UP STRATEGIES •

1. Start today! You're never too old to improve your physical fitness. Never.
2. Focus on the four areas that retard aging: stamina, strength, stretching, and balance.
3. Start small. A few minutes a day will reap enormous rewards.
4. If you can't start today, try to act within the next four days, because acting on any plan within four days is vital to its success.
5. Ask a friend, group, or trainer to hold you accountable. This will increase the likelihood of your sticking to your plan.
6. Listen to music while you exercise to make it more appealing.
7. Add some variety your routine.
8. Walk! It's cheap, local, and simple.
9. Remember that movement lowers stress, which contributes to the number one killer: heart disease.
10. Remember, the more you move, the longer you live.

AGING SUCCESSFULLY: ATTITUDE #8

With proper exercise, I can rekindle and respark my fire for life.

CHAPTER 9

IN THE JAWS OF MENOPAUSE

"Menopause used to be a pit from which many women never emerged...in less than the last five years, we have emerged from the dark ages and moved light years toward a new way of living through and beyond menopause."

—Gail Sheehy, *New Passages*[1]

"There is an appointed time for everything. And there is a time for every event under heaven....[God] *has made everything appropriate in its time."*

—Ecclesiastes 3:1, 11

Dolly Parton, Loretta Lynn, and Tammy Wynette—the brass, sass, and class of country music—are together in a room, talking about their first joint album.

"Loretta: 'Dolly, tell 'em what you wanted to call it.'

"'*Hot Flashes,*' squeals Dolly, sending the three into a paroxysm of one-liners."[2]

Dolly knows her market. Millions of American women will be sweating in the "jaws of menopause" in the next 20 years. Even though I am an eternal optimist, I too am locked into those jaws.

Merriam-Webster's 11th Collegiate Dictionary defines *jaws* as "either of two or more movable parts that open and close for holding or crushing something between them." I refuse to be crushed! I refuse to think of this normal process as the end of my youth, the end of pleasurable sex, or the end of looking or feeling good.

For 50 years, my personal health was excellent. But the first time I experienced heart palpitations, I panicked! My mind screamed, *heart attack*!

Then I started sweating. I diagnosed myself as having an infection somewhere in my body.

Gaining weight made me feel guilty for eating too much of the wrong foods!

These symptoms continued, and new ones appeared. When these signs of aging showed up, dislodging my feelings of youthfulness and drowning me with fear, I decided to research menopause. In *Menopause and Midlife*, the authors write, "Menopause and midlife work in tandem. We might think of menopause as a woman's internal, physical upheaval and midlife as her external, emotional upheaval."[3] I began to understand the changes within my body, and I learned to accept them as part and parcel of the midlife package, not a sentence to a useless existence.

This was not an instantaneous acceptance, however, especially when my symptoms pointed me toward a hysterectomy.

Imprisoned by four sterile walls, I held on to the memory of my husband's warm kiss before he'd left the hospital. I blinked back my tears. Fear clogged my throat. I was afraid that I would lose my femininity during the procedure—that I would no longer feel or look attractive. I feared that much of the meaning I derived from life as a woman and a nurturer—a life giver—would disappear with a slash of the scalpel. The next morning, my favorite lingerie would be traded for a surgical gown. And the feminine fragrance I wore would be replaced with the odor of disinfectants and medication.

But my mood changed from gloom to joy when I remembered that I was not alone in that immaculate hospital room. I had an intimate relationship with Jesus Christ. His peace filled my heart. As I prayed, I could feel Him take some of the fear away and replace it with hope. I knew in my heart that He would be with me in this time of need.

God is not some mystical, impersonal power somewhere out in the universe. He's my best Friend, Savior, and Lord. I have learned to trust Him completely. Being closely connected with God the Father, God the Son, and God the Holy Spirit gave me courage to face major surgery with less fear.

Today, I'm completely healthy, but without God, the anguish of surgery would have left scars. Now, whenever I encounter a new or different problem with aging, I know that Jesus Christ will guide me successfully through it.

• POWER AND CHOICES •

Spiritual and intellectual knowledge gives us power and choices, freeing us to explore what Gail Sheehy has termed "the gateway to a Second Adulthood."[4]

In addition to exploring current thoughts and research on menopause, I made an appointment with my Christian gynecologist, Dr. James C. Upchurch, in Birmingham, Alabama. Sensitive to his patients' needs, he answered all my questions about the "change of life." I want to share with you Dr. Upchurch's professional insights into menopause. Knowing what to expect, what symptoms to look for, and how to manage menopause will enable us to sail more smoothly through the rough seas of "the change."

Though many of Dr. Upchurch's patients first consulted him while he was practicing obstetrics, he has spent the latter half of his 30-year career concentrating exclusively on gynecology. Consequently, an increasing number of his patients are menopausal women.

SHIRLEY: Dr. Upchurch, what are women's concerns as they approach menopause?

DR. UPCHURCH: Women are concerned about aging, hot flashes, night sweats, and changed sexual function. Menopause refers to that point in a woman's life when menstruation stops, usually around age 50. For several months or years prior to menopause, women may experience some episodes of hot flashes, night sweats, and irregular periods, with a lack of ovulation taking place. This is known as perimenopause. But women are interested in relief, not in confusing medical terminology, and I agree. When a woman shows symptoms of estrogen deficiency, she wants reassurance and understanding. My patients describe these changes as "being in the menopause," so I tend to use their terminology.

SHIRLEY: What are some of the symptoms of "being in the menopause"?

DR. UPCHURCH: Symptoms might include loss of energy and motivation, sleeping difficulties, heart palpitations, irregular menstruation or cessation of menstruation,[5] mood swings, and constipation. Some experts suggest that there is no relationship between depression and the menopause. Women know better! All we have to do is ask them; they will say, "Of course, depression comes with menopause!"

Another emotional symptom might logically include a change in the way the woman relates to her family.

Physiologically, in addition to hot flashes lasting one to three minutes (called "the hallmark symptom of menopause," and occurring in 50 to 75 percent of women[6]), night sweats can interrupt a woman's sleep, making her tired and irritable. A menopausal woman might also experience vaginal dryness, urinary incontinence, sagging breasts, hair changes, osteoporosis, aging or dry skin, and a loss or lowering of her sex drive.

When any of these symptoms occur, the woman should insist upon a sensitive, adequate discussion of the menopause and request a follicle-stimulating hormone blood test from her doctor. If that test reveals that she is menopausal, then she and her physician can discuss adequate hormone management. It is vital that the woman establish good communication with her doctor. Adjustments of the hormones are usually fairly simple, but sometimes numerous dosages and hormone types may have to be tried.

SHIRLEY: We know that proper exercise and diet help women manage some of the side effects of menopause, but what is the best available medical management of menopause?

DR. UPCHURCH: Most menopausal patients benefit from estrogen. Menopause is brought about by the lowering of estrogen, produced by the ovaries. Because many symptoms of menopause are the result of these lower estrogen levels, with estrogen replacement, many symptoms are reduced or eliminated.

In addition to estrogen, women should take 1000–1500 mg of calcium per day, with vitamin D added to better metabolize the calcium.

Beyond controlling symptoms of menopause, estrogen has other beneficial effects.

SHIRLEY: What are some of those benefits of estrogen?

DR. UPCHURCH: Estrogen locks calcium in the bones. Osteoporosis—the condition where the bones lose calcium, become thin, and break easily—results from loss of calcium in the bones and affects 50 percent of women after menopause. Estrogen replacement therapy (ERT) will stop the bone loss, especially when calcium, vitamin D, and exercise are used. It is reversed by increasing a woman's estrogen levels.[7]

Estrogen also protects the coronary arteries from clogging with fat deposits. Estrogens have been shown to reduce the mortality rate from coronary artery disease at a rate of 50 percent by age 65. Thousands of women are spared coronary deaths because they started estrogen replacement at the onset of menopause.

Also, studies show that the incidence of Alzheimer's is reduced by about 40 percent when estrogens are used regularly.

SHIRLEY: What other benefits might women expect from taking estrogen supplements?

DR. UPCHURCH: Estrogen helps to decrease vaginal dryness, improve the skin and hair, and restore more normal sleep patterns. There is also a sense of well-being in a patient on estrogen, an increased quality of life that cannot be defined scientifically. A patient may well say, "I feel like myself again."

Often, just a slight increase in a hormone dosage makes a tremendous difference in the way a patient feels, both psychologically and physically.

There is no doubt in my mind that depression, fatigue, and the ability to cope are significantly altered by a little drop in hormone and are improved dramatically by an increase in medication.

SHIRLEY: While we're talking about estrogen, what are some of the disadvantages to estrogen supplements? For instance, does estrogen cause phlebitis (blood clots)?

DR. UPCHURCH: Research shows that the incidence of deep vein phlebitis (DVT) is increased in estrogen users.[8] The usual incidence of DVT is about one to two cases per 10,000 women; estrogen treatment increases this to three to four per 10,000 women. Women over 60 with *known* heart disease should be warned that there is an increase in phlebitis and heart attacks if they are taking estrogen for the first time.

Gallstone development is slightly more likely with ERT. An increase in asthma attacks has also been reported with ERT.

SHIRLEY: What if a woman has a history of phlebitis (blood clotting), pulmonary emboli, or stroke, and she is taking blood thinners?

DR. UPCHURCH: Women with these disorders probably shouldn't take estrogen,[9] though estrogen is compatible with virtually every medication, including blood thinners. Women taking blood thinners for coagulation problems should have their clotting time monitored more frequently if on estrogen because estrogen may make the blood thinner even more effective, thus lengthening the clotting time. Such patients need to be followed by a hematologist if estrogen is felt to be advisable. Women with protein S deficiency and similar diseases shouldn't use estrogen, because phlebitis is a very high possibility.

SHIRLEY: Besides women with known heart disease and clotting problems, should all other menopausal women take estrogens?

DR. UPCHURCH: Women with breast cancer traditionally do not take estrogen, although some five- and ten-year survivors take estrogens.

SHIRLEY: What about the breast cancer scare? Do hormones increase the risk of breast cancer?

DR. UPCHURCH: A few studies[10] have shown an increase in the incidence of breast cancer in certain groups, but most studies do not show a statistically significant increase. Considering the prevalence of heart disease over cancer of any kind,[11] the benefits of estrogen to the heart outweigh any minimal risk of breast cancer, in my opinion.

Current prevailing opinion is that even women with a family history of breast cancer should take estrogen because of the vast benefits, assuming that they are being monitored by a doctor because of their family history. Should tumors occur, women taking estrogen, on the average, usually have a lower grade malignancy in their tumors.

SHIRLEY: What about women with fibrocystic breast disease?

DR. UPCHURCH: Fibrocystic breast disease is not really a disease but more a glandular change in the breast that causes some discomfort and lumpiness. It is not a precancerous process. Sometimes estrogen increases the discomfort and tenderness of the breast.

Some physicians prefer that patients with severe fibrocystic change not use estrogens. These women should follow the advice of their physician. In our practice, we like our fibrocystic-change patients to have regular mammograms and regular examinations; some need consultation with a surgeon.

At times, a patient becomes very difficult to evaluate because of the lumpiness. The surgeon might recommend the discontinuation of the estrogen preparations, but this is unusual.

SHIRLEY: What about a woman who has had breast augmentation (implants)? Would estrogen present any problems for her?

DR. UPCHURCH: It's harder to diagnose lesions in a woman with breast augmentation, but taking estrogen isn't any riskier for her.

SHIRLEY: Are there women in the menopausal age range who do not need estrogen?

DR. UPCHURCH: Some patients feel fine throughout the menopausal changes and do not want to take estrogens. However, these women will still need estrogen, for the reasons already discussed.

SHIRLEY: When should a woman begin ERT or hormone replacement therapy?

DR. UPCHURCH: She should begin at the first signs of menopause. There are women who have had both the uterus and ovaries removed (called an oophorectomy) and abruptly become hormone deficient. This is called surgical menopause, and these women usually need hormone treatment immediately after surgery. Most surgical menopause women have severe symptoms unless treated with estrogen replacement.

SHIRLEY: What hormones are available to the menopausal woman?

DR. UPCHURCH: Women during the reproductive years produce three different estrogen hormones from the ovaries: estradiol, estrone, and estriol.

Progesterone is also produced, and it brings about menstrual bleeding by causing about two thirds of the uterine lining to break off. The ovaries also produce androgens (a group of male hormones which include testosterone) in small amounts.

In the reproductive years, the female hormone estradiol is by far the most powerful and has the most profound effect upon the lining of the uterus.

Of *oral estrogens*, one of the most popular hormones is the conjugated estrogens hormone derived from pregnant mares' urine, which circulates in the blood primarily as estrone. This hormone has been available the longest and is the one most studied. It has definitely been shown to be very effective in reducing cholesterol in the bloodstream, especially the bad cholesterol (LDL). It has also been shown to protect the coronary arteries and is effective in treating osteoporosis. In appropriate dosages, this estrogen works nicely in diminishing or eliminating menopausal symptoms.

Along with conjugated estrogens, estradiol tablets are available. They have had less study than conjugated estrogens, but are probably equivalent protection against osteoporosis and coronary artery disease development.

An alternative to oral estrogens is *transdermal estrogen*, found in the estradiol skin patch. (The patch is also available with both estrogen and progesterone.) Each patch lasts either three-and-a-half or seven days, and then it must be replaced. Estrogen is absorbed through the skin from the patch, usually on the buttocks or abdomen, into the arterial system. It circulates much like the normal estrogen output from the ovaries.

With the patch, unfortunately, many patients report skin irritation, sometimes so severe that they discontinue the patch, even though the patch alleviates their menopausal symptoms.

Intramuscular injections of estradiol are another possibility; they are given monthly.

Estradiol *pellets*, another alternative, may be inserted under the abdominal skin through a small incision with a special applicator. The pellet is made of compressed estradiol crystals, which circulate into the arterial system. The pellet lasts approximately three to six months, then dissolves. One disadvantage of this method is that, once inserted, the pellet cannot be removed, should the patient not respond well to the treatment.

Another disadvantage is that a small incision is made each time the pellet is inserted, leaving some small scars over the lower abdominal skin. I use this technique for women who have not been able to take their estrogen successfully any other way.

Occasionally, when a patient reports significant fatigue, lack of energy, and lack of sexual libido, I insert a testosterone pellet. Patients often report beneficial effects from this therapy. However, testosterone may offset the cardiovascular benefits of estradiol, so I'd rather not prescribe testosterone pellets. Monitoring the patient's cholesterol levels is essential. Overdoses of testosterone can cause weight gain; increased muscle mass; enhanced appetite; coarse, oily skin with acne; and an enlarged clitoris. Testosterone is the hormone that induces facial hair growth and a permanent lowering of the voice.

SHIRLEY: What about combined hormone replacement therapy?

DR. UPCHURCH: Some oral medications contain a testosterone in combination with estrogen. These compounds are not recommended for long-term use.

But typical hormone replacement therapy refers to estrogen and progesterone combinations; these are available in tablets and in skin patches. Patients who still have their uterus must take progesterone as well as estrogen. Estrogen without progesterone increases the risk of uterine (endometrial) cancer.

I do not prescribe progesterone cream, which patients rub into their skin, usually on the arms or thighs. Estrogens and progesterones compounded by the local pharmacy are becoming more readily available, but I am not prescribing them. There are no large studies to convince me to change from the medications that have served my patients so well for many years.

One disadvantage of adding progesterone is that, depending on the dosage and the form of administration, it may result in the return of the "periods" and even PMS. If administered cyclically, with estrogen given alone in the first half of the month and then progesterone added in the second half of the cycle, bleeding may occur. Combined dosage of both hormones will often prevent this.

SHIRLEY: If a patient does not take estrogens, can she take a satisfactory substitute?

DR. UPCHURCH: There is a category of medications known as selective estrogen receptor modulators (SERMS), which will help prevent osteoporosis when used with calcium supplementation. These compounds probably also reduce the incidence of breast cancer, but they may not protect the coronary arteries. If a patient cannot or will not take estrogens, then she should use a SERM to help prevent bone loss.

SHIRLEY: Menopause surely affects the woman; it just as surely impacts the man in her life, as well! I remember those night sweats, when I'd have to change the sheets in the middle of the night. What advice do you give men whose wives are in menopause, Dr. Upchurch?

DR. UPCHURCH: Husbands are not always sensitive about the changes of the menopause because they are uninformed. It's a good idea for the husband, wife, and doctor to meet together to discuss some of these changes. The husband needs to understand the mental, physical, and psychological changes of his wife.

After all, when wedding vows are exchanged, a couple promises to stay married, in sickness and in health, until death. Young fathers are permitted to be present during labor and delivery, even coaching their wives through the miraculous birth of their children. Likewise, a husband needs to come alongside his wife during these years of menopause; she not only needs his compassion and understanding–she deserves it.

• QUESTIONS FOR IMMEDIATE APPLICATION •

1. After reading the interview with Dr. Upchurch, write down three ways you will open those "jaws of menopause" in your own life.
2. List any questions related to menopause you desire to ask your own doctor.
3. Some people believe that truly "spiritual" women won't need hormone replacement therapy. How do you feel about this? Why?
4. If you are married, how will you share with your husband the changes you are experiencing, the help you are receiving for any problems, and your optimism for a renewed, exciting sex life with him?
5. Be active, not passive: create an action plan for dealing with menopause. Include all areas: emotional, physical, spiritual, and relational.

• TOP TEN PERIMENOPAUSE/ MENOPAUSE STRATEGIES •

1. Learn the symptoms of (peri)menopause.

2. List the advantages of menopause. (It's a challenge, but do it, anyway.)
3. Face your concerns about aging, specifically menopause.
4. Find a compassionate doctor who will work with you through the treatment options to make the most of menopause. Get an estrogen-level blood test and a bone density test.
5. Figure out together what you can do physically (through exercise, diet modification, stress reduction, etc.) to make this passage easier.
6. If you are married, talk with your husband about the emotional and physical changes you are experiencing. Bring him along the next time you see your doctor.
7. Know your family history: cancer, heart disease, your mother's age at the onset of menopause, and so forth.
8. Slim down your calendar of commitments. Big transitions, such as menopause, drain your emotional and physical energy. Plan to take care of yourself during this time.
9. Surround yourself with supportive people.
10. Be tenacious. This is your life and your body. Ask questions. Keep asking until you get answers that work for you.

AGING SUCCESSFULLY: ATTITUDE #9

I will open the jaws of menopause with help from my doctor, healthy habits, and a great attitude.

CHAPTER 10

FIFTYISH–FEMALE–FABULOUS

"A person who has good thoughts cannot ever be ugly. You can have a wonky nose and a crooked mouth and a double chin and stick-out teeth, but if you have good thoughts they will shine out of your face like sunbeams and you will always look lovely."

–Roald Dahl, The Twits[1]

"Now you're dressed in a new wardrobe. Every item of your new way of life is custom-made by the Creator, with his label on it. All the old fashions are now obsolete....So, chosen by God for this new life of love, dress in the wardrobe God picked out for you: compassion, kindness, humility, quiet strength, discipline....And regardless of what else you put on, wear love. It's your basic, all-purpose garment. Never be without it."

–Colossians 3:9–14 (MSG)

The banner's shiny, black background accentuated the hot pink words, which screamed, "Fiftyish! Female! Fabulous!" Beneath the flamboyant banner, the Writers' Roundtable Critique Group had gathered excitedly, ready to celebrate my 50th birthday.

"Shirley, your passage to the second half-century of life is paving the way for me. I don't think I will be depressed," my author friend Gay Martin author of *Alabama Off the Beaten Path* and *Louisiana Off the Beaten Path*, told me with a big hug. "Can you believe it? With the aging baby boomer, 50-something is in vogue!"

The group laughed, grateful to be in such "fashionable" company.

My thoughts raced back to the morning I had spoken at the Thursday Study Club, an elite group in my hometown, about being "50ish, female, and fabulous." That talk had proven to be Motivation with a capital "M"! I have discovered that it takes attention and creativity to be spiffy at 50: attention to hair, skin, and clothing, as well as to diet and exercise, and menopause management.

• HAIR CARE •

Hair is supposed to be the crown of our appearance; unfortunately, our hormones don't always cooperate. Menopause can make hair dry, brittle, and sparse. Helped along by hormone replacement therapy (HRT), our hair can make a comeback.

Our "crown" starts with a hairstyle suitable for our face shape. In general, a hairstyle should not duplicate one's face shape. A woman with a rounded face should avoid a hairstyle that repeats that roundness. She might opt for a style that creates some angles around her jaw line. Long hair with no bangs emphasizes a long face; bangs or a gentle feathering across the brow would create emphasis and horizontal interest.

Fortunately, a daring new cut or color needn't be risky at all, thanks to the computer imaging techniques available in many salons today. A current picture is all that the hairstylist needs to allow the customer to "try on" a new look—without any cutting or coloring.

Too many women make the mistake of believing that long hair always equals youthful appearance. While long hair does cover the aging neck, it can also draw the face down. A great hairstyle should draw attention to the eyes, where the soul shines through.

Some women may choose to cover their gray; others opt for natural. The most basic rule is to match hair color with skin tones. When Carole Jackson's book *Color Me Beautiful* appeared on the scene in the late 1970s, the principles of selecting which color to wear and dye our hair suddenly made sense.[2] For example, a blue undertone in the skin truly makes red hair a poor choice; yellow undertones with dyed black hair can make us look sickly. For best results, color choices should be made with the expertise of a reputable stylist.

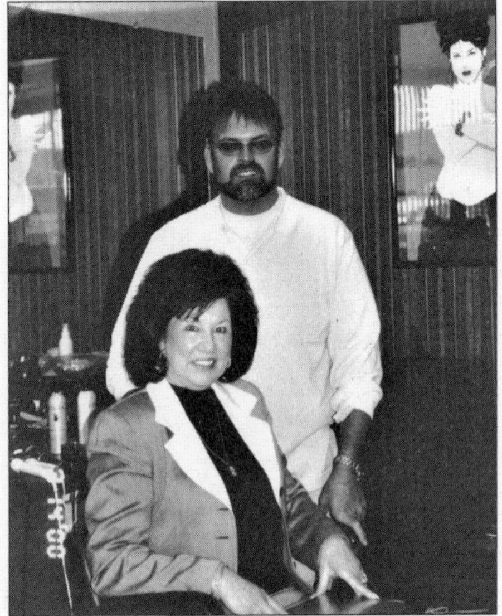

Shirley with Michael King, her hairstylist

Some options for hair color include:

Glossers—these add sheen and shine with little or no color.

Full Color—never exceed two levels lighter than your natural color.

Highlights—if you are in the natural blonde family, choose a lighter shade to complement your own color. Lowlights add tones and dimension to brunettes and redheads.

Semipermanent Tint—adds tone to natural hair without commitment, if you are just starting to gray.

Increased volume can be accomplished by using professional products at the root area and learning the art of blow-drying. This is preferable to the old "teasing" technique (properly called backcombing), which takes thin hair and poofs it up. Finishing products add shine to the completed style.

Beautiful hair is a crown to our appearance, and posture is a crown to self-assurance and a confident air.

• POSTURE •

Studying my wedding pictures, I noticed that, as a 20-year-old woman, I practiced perfect posture. Now that I am fabulous after 50, perfect posture is not spontaneous. I must make a conscious effort to practice good posture.

When I slump, my shoulders round, and a ledge of fat accumulates around my waist. I literally must stand tall to look younger. Good bones help me stand tall, too.

Though our bodies are not perfect, we can stand tall and portray an individualistic, elegant look, with a body language that says, "I'm making the most of myself and my life." Proper posture takes years off our age and generates respect—and often a second look!—from others. Looking in a mirror, we'll also find that our clothes look better when we stand up straight.

It helps to be able to see ourselves in that mirror, however, to make the most of the best!

• EYESIGHT •

Until I was 40, I enjoyed 20/20 vision. After 40, my arms got too short for me to find a number in the telephone directory. Thank the Lord for contact lenses!

One friend, Lynn, kept her paperwork constantly moving in front of her until she found the precise distance at which she could read the print. She held off getting an eye exam because, she said, "I look terrible in glasses." Finally, after trying on reading glasses at the pharmacy, she settled on a nonthreatening pair and has fully adjusted to her new fashion tool.

If eyeglasses are in the picture for you, the same rule for hairstyles applies: do not repeat the shape of your face or the shape of your jawline in your eyeglasses. Round rims on a round face will make you look like you're ready to roll away. Go for contrast—create some opposing lines for interest.

Also, avoid tinted glasses for inside wear; not only are they quickly dated, but they rarely match skin tone. Nonglare lenses make it easier for others to look you in the eye and don't reflect the camera flash in photographs.

With eyes to see, we are ready to look in the mirror—a well-lighted one, of course! If you don't have good light in your bathroom, consider buying a special mirror with suction cups that will adhere to the window, so that you may study yourself in the natural illumination of daylight.

• SKIN CARE •

A good skin care regime starts with a revitalizing mask to exfoliate dead surface cells. You should choose a mask appropriate to your skin type, whether dry or oily. And, because skin changes with menopause, you may need to adjust the moisturizer in your skin care routine.

Drinking eight glasses of water a day keeps skin firm-looking and youthful; just as a plant droops without water, so our skin withers if it isn't properly hydrated. My sister, Debra Goodwin, contrasts well-hydrated skin with an apple that has sat on the counter for days and is shrunken and shriveled. Water in our system plumps our skin! What an easy addition to our daily agenda.

I follow my facial mask with a toner to leave my skin refreshed and revitalized.

Scrutiny in the mirror may also reveal those dreaded age spots. Dermatologists can help lighten them, but more will appear as we age. Sun, often the culprit of age spots, finally caught up with me. Working in the cotton fields with my dad until I was 18 took its toll on my skin! Dabbing some tinted concealer on age spots minimizes their appearance.

We should invest in products containing sunscreen, which protects our face and neck from the sun. When we follow this with a moisturizer and a thin layer of liquid foundation, our faces will glow with health! Be certain to look closely in that mirror now, because a makeup line forming a boundary along the jaw adds years to the appearance. By blending foundation underneath the jawbone and onto the neck, we avoid this age-amplifier. Go easy, too, on the layered look; makeup that is thick enough to scrape off is a dead giveaway of the desperate aging woman.

Glamour comes next, as we apply makeup to emphasize eyes, cheekbones, and lips. My daughter, Karen Corcoran, a consultant for Mary Kay Cosmetics, has taught me the art of applying eye shadow, eyeliner, and lush eyelash extender to make my small, set-back eyes appear large and expressive. Rouge, or blush, and lipstick should be selected to complement skin tone, hair, and clothing. To avoid a dated makeup look, a trip to your favorite cosmetician for a makeover is a lovely lift.

• KEY FASHION RULES •

Understanding the function of lines is important when deciding how to dress. Our eyes tend to follow every line, and to stop where a line ends. Horizontal lines add width; vertical lines add height. Lines create emphasis, so we never want to end a line at our widest point. For instance, a jacket should not stop at the widest part of your hip. Hem length should emphasize the best part of your leg, not necessarily your wide calves! The large-busted woman should avoid lines or patterns in the bust area, as details always add weight.

Details can be used appropriately, however, to create balance. Pockets on the rear round out a flat derriere; pockets, gathers, or stripes along the bust line create the illusion of a more buxom woman. Emphasizing our best features, and minimizing those we aren't as fond of, makes it easier to be other-directed. As we discover our personal style and find the clothes we're comfortable in, we will dress for successful aging.

• YOUR OWN PERSONAL STYLE •

Individual taste, lifestyle, and body shape will determine the style of chic wrappings you will choose to best demonstrate your unique persona and beauty. As we age, we need not automatically assume the guise of dowdy housewife or frump. "Dressing our age" should refer not only to our body type but also to our spirit! This doesn't mean dressing girlishly and looking foolish;

it does mean taking into account both our body type and our personality.

Creating the look we desire can be fun and rewarding, and it needn't involve revamping our entire wardrobe and going into debt! Department stores employ professional sales associates who are trained to help patrons find the right garments and accessories for them. In addition, starting with some basic foundational garments multiplies our options.

For one of the Miss America pageants, all 50 contestants were dressed in a basic black dress, a fashion essential for every woman. Unique accessories gave each contestant a splash of color. As the 50 girls danced and twirled around the stage, I observed the versatility of the smart black dress. We can dress it up, dress it down, cover it with a cape, accessorize it, wear a jacket over it—the possibilities are limitless!

If black is not your best neutral color, figure out which one is. Neutrals include navy, brown, beige, bone, and winter white, in addition to black. Building a wardrobe around the single best neutral for our skin tones means that our shoes will always match, and we can use colored accessories to enhance the ensemble.

Making color work for us helps us feel dazzling, brings new life to our skin and face, and draws attention upward to our eyes. Don't be afraid of color; color says, "I am confident!" Knowing our underlying skin tone, we are free to focus on which hues and colors look best on us.

Our role model from God's Word, "*the virtuous woman*" (Proverbs 31:10 KJV) made her clothing of fine linen and purple, and clothed her family in scarlet. (See Proverbs 31:21–22 NIV.) Her clothing reflected her confident lifestyle, as well as the brilliance of her Creator.

Like the beautiful girls in the Miss America Pageant, and like our Proverbs 31 woman, clothes can make us dance, cause our mood to leap to new heights, and give us a sense of adventure.

As for accessories, less is more. Too many details can confuse the casual observer. An understated presentation of carefully selected jewelry or a scarf, emphasizing our best features, presents a powerful, put-together image. Whatever our clothing personality, we can run toward our Goliath of aging in great style.

I wrote the following poem to remind myself of a basic truth:

I want to be the best that I can be!
All that God's created in me.
Like someone else I cannot be.
I just want to be me.

Whether we are speaking to an elite study group or moving confidently ahead in other arenas, by putting our best image forward, wrapping ourselves in an aura of passion, and sparkling with love and an interest in others, we put ourselves in the winners' circle.

• QUESTIONS FOR IMMEDIATE APPLICATION •

1. Give three reasons 50-something is in vogue. What is one word that best describes your personality and your sense of style? Elegant? Natural? Tomboy?
2. If you could "dress your age and your spirit," what would you wear? A long flowing dress? Crop-top and cutoffs? Denim? Silk? List five ways you will be the best you can be, now.
3. What would the "winners' circle" look like to you? Write out a personal profile describing the steps you will take to put yourself in the winners' circle in the last half of your life.

• TOP TEN FABULOUS FASHION STRATEGIES •

1. Even if nobody seems to talk about it anymore, find out which colors work bets on you. You'll never regret wearing them.
2. After that, start at the top, with your hair and face shape, and work your way down. What lines look best where?
3. Figure out where you need to create width or height, and then determine which styles will do that for you.
4. Measure your widest points and determine not to end lines in those locations.
5. Clean out your closet and then reorganize it by color and type of clothing item.
6. Go to your favorite makeup counter and get a makeover. Be sure to ask for complimentary samples.
7. Remember, looking good gives the God who created you all the glory. Who needs dowdy?
8. Don't assume you should wear a certain item just because it looks good on someone else. Style is defined by your life, your passion, and your personality–not by emaciated and grim-faced models on the runway.
9. Remember that body changes are inevitable, and no one has a perfect body. (Marilyn Monroe was a size 14.) Stop pining away for the body you once had, never had, or wish you had, and get on with taking care of the one you're currently inhabiting.
10. When you finally know that you look your best, forget yourself and focus on others.

AGING SUCCESSFULLY: ATTITUDE #10

To be 50ish, female, and fabulous, I will make the most of my best.

CHAPTER 11

AN EXCITING AND VIBRANT LIFE FROM HERE TO ETERNITY

"I want to experience the pleasure of knowing God with greater intensity as I age. I want my soul to become skilled and comfortable in the practice of heaven–praising and enjoying God. I'm acclimating my eternal soul, my intrinsic self, to the values of heaven now."

Valerie Bell, *She Can Laugh at the Days to Come*[1]

"I will fulfill the number of your days."

–Exodus 23:26

As I pulled my car out of my driveway, I praised God for my wonderful life. En route to a lecture at Snead State College, I picked up my friend Gay Martin. We chatted nonstop through the sunshine and the traffic. Pulling up to a red light, I braked, checking my rearview mirror to see if the truck behind me had stopped, as well. It had. Confident, I glanced again at Gay.

Suddenly, my car lunged forward, my door caved in, and the rearview mirror was ripped off. The windshield shattered into a million pieces, and the car was tossed off the road. The crumbling of chrome, steel, and glass was deafening.

Astounded that we were not hurt, Gay and I crawled from the wreckage with trembling limbs and turned to see what had crashed into us. Another semi, directly behind the first 18-wheeler, had been unable to stop and tried to maneuver between my car and the vehicle stopped next to me at the red light.

An amazing sense of God's presence and protection filled my heart, along with a new awareness of how fragile life is. With that awareness came the sense that we are always just one breath away from eternity. I praised God that He had allowed me to stay on this earth a short time longer, before my street turned to gold.

• ETERNITY NOW •

My brush with death has given me a sense of heaven in the here and now. For this reason alone, aging is not a negative! The Scripture says, "*Take hold of the eternal life to which you were called*" (1 Timothy 6:12). In this way, aging becomes an even greater opportunity to embrace possibility.

In church on New Year's Day, 1996, the year the baby boom generation approached the threshold of 50, I looked at the cover of the sermon bulletin, a vivid picture that caught my attention. Sticking up out of the snow, a new, bright-colored flower grew straight and tall, stretching toward the sun. The snow could not hinder it. The picture shouted to my spirit: "New life! New beginning!"

The big, bold, colorful words at the top of the picture shot into my soul, as straight as an arrow: "*Behold, I make all things new*" (Revelation 21:5 KJV).

In the spirit of reflection that accompanies the start of each new year, I enjoyed my own private inventory of the past. My mind also exploded with ideas, dreams, possibilities, and hopes for the future. During my quiet time that New Year's Day, I meditated on the entirety of that verse passage from Revelation: *"He that sat upon the throne said, Behold, I make all things new. And he said unto me, Write: for these words are true and faithful"* (Revelation 21:5 KJV) In this verse, God was speaking to the apostle John, the writer of the book of Revelation.

However, to me, also a writer, this Scripture spoke volumes about my future. As I make plans and pray through them, I rejoice in this perennial hopefulness, which pushes past frigid barriers and shoots for the sun.

When Christ says, *"I make all things new,"* He not only means you and me; He means everything: aging, our understanding of our value in His sight, our purpose in life, and even death. In death we learn, ultimately, that life is forever.

• LIFE IS FOREVER •

Life is spirit, not just flesh and blood; therefore, with Jesus Christ as our Savior, Master, and Lord, we embrace death because, in death, we find our true selves—we are freed at last from our old human form to a body capable of living for all eternity. Our lives are consumed in the process of growing up into all the fullness of God (see Ephesians 3:19), and at death, we will finally be like Him, for we shall see Him as He is. (See 1 John 3:2.)

Death laid a soft blanket of peace over my friend, who had been trapped for four years in a body that did not work. In death, as in life, she appeared in control. In the twinkling of an eye, she inhabited a new body and entered through the pearly gates. Years before this date, she had chosen to be born again, into the kingdom of God. She had made her reservation years in advance!

Lou Gehrig's disease was not big enough to amputate her spirit. In health and in sickness, her spirit remained the same—bright, big, and magnificent.

She had preplanned the celebration of her memorial service. Being a superb hostess in life, she proved to be even better in death. I've always known that life can be magical; during that final celebration of her passing, I experienced that magic. The encouraging words from the people of God, the Bible, and the heavenly music lifted my spirit to the heights of heaven. Her preplanning indicated her great faith and longing for her real home.

• OUR REAL HOME •

"The trees, like the longings of the earth, stand a-tiptoe to peep at the heaven," said Sir Rabindranath Tagore.[2] Like the trees, fabulous-after-50 women desire a peep into heaven, our real home. We are, after all, only a heartbeat away from there.

Our all-knowing God knew we would be curious about our future home, so He gives us a glimpse of heaven in His Holy Bible:

> *One of the seven angels...came and said to me, "Come, I will show you the bride, the wife of the Lamb." And he carried me away in the Spirit to a mountain great and high, and showed me the Holy City, Jerusalem, coming down out of heaven from God. It shone with the glory of God, and its brilliance was like that of a very precious jewel, like a jasper, clear as crystal. It had a great, high wall with twelve gates, and with twelve angels at the gates. On the gates were written the names of the twelve tribes of Israel. There were three gates on the east, three on the north, three on the south and three on the west. The wall of the city had twelve foundations, and on them were the names of the twelve apostles of the Lamb. The angel who*

talked with me had a measuring rod of gold to measure the city, its gates and its walls. The city was laid out like a square, as long as it was wide. He measured the city with the rod and found it to be 12,000 stadia in length, and as wide and high as it is long. He measured its wall and it was 144 cubits thick, by man's measurement, which the angel was using. The wall was made of jasper, and the city of pure gold, as pure as glass. The foundations of the city walls were decorated with every kind of precious stone. The first foundation was jasper, the second sapphire, the third chalcedony, the fourth emerald, the fifth sardonyx, the sixth carnelian, the seventh chrysolite, the eighth beryl, the ninth topaz, the tenth chrysoprase, the eleventh jacinth, and the twelfth amethyst. The twelve gates were twelve pearls, each gate made of a single pearl. The great street of the city was of pure gold, like transparent glass.

(Revelation 21:9–21 NIV)

Life's imperfections and strivings are only a prelude to the perfection of heaven, highlighting our longing for that completion.

• THE WEDDING •

I have attended some beautiful weddings. The gorgeous brides and their many helpers worked for months to perfect every detail. A radiant bride is the most beautiful sight on earth. I think the glorious perfection of heaven must be a perfect wedding multiplied a zillion times.

Included in that perfection will be total communication, ultimate good, and living in the presence of God.

We can only imagine the intensity and joy of a life where there is no death, sorrow, crying, or pain. (See Revelation 21:4.) The crowning moment is being in the presence of Jesus.

My worship time each morning of Holy Week 2000 was a glorious meditation as I gazed upon a painting by famous artist William Hallmark entitled *The Bride of Christ*. The piece depicts the artist's rendering of Revelation 19:7, "*Let us rejoice and be glad and give him glory! For the wedding of the Lamb has come, and his bride has made herself ready*" (NIV). I saw the bride of Christ through the artist's eyes. The glory of Christ shone forth from the face of the radiant bride, dressed in dazzling white and watching out a window. Jesus, transparent, standing behind her, looking down upon her, seemed to whisper, "I will be your husband." Both of their ring fingers were touching, each one bearing a wedding band. The feeling that Jesus is my Husband flooded my heart and I longed for God to shine His glory—His *shekinah* glory—through my face and life.

• HEAVEN NOW •

Meditating on heaven during my daily walk that afternoon, still trembling from my earlier accident, I watched dying embers of the day turn the clouds into brilliant goldas the setting sun dropped over the horizon like a fiery ball.

Diverting my eyes from the magnificent sunset, I looked to the east and beheld a gorgeous full moon, plastered against an azure sky. An airplane cut a path across the surface of the moon, makings its descent into our small town's airport.

As I looked west toward the brilliant rays of the sunset, a group of birds flying in perfect synchronized precision caught my attention.

My ears picked up the sounds of life—children laughing while playing, dogs barking, tractors plowing, cows mooing, birds singing.

The fragrance of honeysuckle perfumed the cool evening air. I breathed deeply, filling my healthy lungs.

The breathing exercise brought tears to my eyes as I remembered the semi truck and my brush with death. Just one breath away from eternity.

Joy filled my soul, much like the air had filled my lungs, and I praised God for allowing me to experience this magnificent evening, joyfully soaking my soul with the beauty of life.

This feeling of praise widens to cover the past half century of my life—and the next one! Hallelujah! It's fabulous to be 50!

• QUESTIONS FOR IMMEDIATE APPLICATION •

1. Knowing that we are spiritual beings, and that, through Jesus Christ, we will live eternally, how do you feel about death?
2. Knowing you are moving daily toward eternity, how will you appreciate, anticipate, enjoy, and fill each day of your mature life?
3. What is your vision of heaven?

• TOP TEN THINGS TO LOOK FORWARD TO IN HEAVEN •

1. Throw away the hankies! No more death, sorrow, tears, or pain! (See Revelation 21:4.)
2. We get a new body! "*We shall also bear the image of the heavenly.... We will all be changed,....This mortal must put on immortality*" (1 Corinthians 15:49–53).
3. No more mortgage payments! Jesus said, "*I go and prepare a place for you*" (John 14:3).

4. No more taxes! The streets are paved with God's gold, not ours.
5. No more standby flights—we get a quick trip! "*For the Lord himself will descend from heaven with a shout,....Then we who are alive and remain shall be caught up...in the clouds to meet the Lord in the air, and thus we shall always be with the Lord*" (1 Thessalonians 4:16–17).
6. We have a constant companion: "*The Father...will give you another Helper* [the Holy Spirit], *that He may be with you forever*" (John 14:16).
7. No more tension headaches. Jesus left us a great gift: "*Peace I leave with you; My peace I give to you; not as the world gives do I give to you. Let not your heart be troubled, nor let it be fearful*" (John 14:27).
8. While waiting for eternity, observe this instruction: "*A new commandment I give to you, that you love one another, even as I have loved you*" (John 13:34).
9. We have a calling! "*Walk in a manner worthy of the God who calls you into His own kingdom and glory*" (1 Thessalonians 2:12).
10. Eternity starts now! "*Take hold now of the eternal life to which you were called*" (1 Timothy 6:12). Be fabulous after 50 forever!

AGING SUCCESSFULLY: ATTITUDE #11

I will dance with anticipation every day of my life as I move toward eternity and my final home.

CHAPTER 12

SIZZLING WITH SIGNIFICANCE

One year, at the National Religious Broadcasters' Convention at the Opryland in Nashville, Tennessee, I parked myself in the center of the Exhibit Hall to observe all of the fabulous, 50-years-young women in attendance.

Wow! Charismatic women who had lived half a century certainly gave me a positive role model. Two fabulous-after-50 women swished passed me in their stilettos, leaving a sweet fragrance of lavender in the air. They were walking briskly, talking, and laughing, their briefcases swinging in their hands. These fearless, fun females were simply ageless. Their passion for their television careers and for broadcasting the gospel was evident in their body language. Their appearance radiated the aura of a star! Christian women are God's stars in our world. Observing these fabulous 50-year-old women, I understood the passion they had for God, life, and their aging future. Passion is one key to being fabulous after 50.

Pushing through the turnstile in 50th year of life is a jubilee for women. The half-century mark is the time to live large, and living large is infectious!

Fifty-year-old females have different stages and agendas. Many of them are the heart of their homes, and have raised beautiful, happy, healthy children. Their families have become God's masterpieces. These successful mothers are seeing their beloved children become independent adults embarking on their own journeys. Although they leave home, their family ties remain strong, and grandchildren strengthen the wonderful feeling of belonging to one other.

Excitement for life continues after 50 for those who dare it to. The "fabulous 50" birthday celebration should last for the rest of our life. Maddy Kent Dychtwald, a member of Age Wave, Inc., stated at a recent conference, "Contrary to popular opinion, there is life after youth, and life can be good!" She believes Americans will change their standard of measure from number of years to life stages.

With positive life experiences, good health, and healthy ambition, age 50 can be the zenith of a woman's life, if she has grown into her God-given adult self. She is the first lady of her own life, standing in the middle of her life stage with Jesus. Hopefully, she has taken her faith to center stage with her. This milestone is a thrilling time in her lifecycle! The love of God and family gives her wings to fly higher into the wind currents of life. She is as an eagle, rising above the difficult times in life. A godly woman is blessed with joy and a positive attitude. She will be an inspiration to others when they go through hard times.

King Solomon wrote, "*The fear of the* L*ORD is the beginning of wisdom: and the knowledge of the holy is understanding. For by me thy days shall be multiplied, and the years of thy life shall be increased*" (Proverbs 9:10–11 KJV).

You can increase the days of your life by looking good, feeling good, and doing good.

• LOOKING GOOD •

When you feel in your heart that you look your best, you shine forth an aura of beauty and self-confidence. Have you ever made a quick trip to the grocery store with a raincoat over your pajamas to grab an item you needed for a recipe? Did you lower you head and walk briskly through the grocery aisles without speaking to anyone because you were embarrassed? Appearance is important to a woman, and it greatly affects her ability to communicate with the people God puts in her path.

When I was a young bride, my groom was a spontaneous person. He would call on the phone and invite me to travel with him to Birmingham, Alabama, and then hop a plane to attend a meeting in Washington, D.C. After missing out on a few exciting lunch dates or trips because I didn't feel fit to be seen, I vowed that my routine would be to get out of bed and dress for success, no matter what the day brought forth. I have followed that plan for a half century, and life has been full of pizzazz!

God created women to be beautiful! Most women are at least mildly interested in fashion, makeup, style, shoes, radiance, and charm. Powder your face with the sunshine of a smile, and pull those shoulders back as you walk with great posture, holding your head high and remembering that you are royalty. God is your heavenly Father!

I am continually impressed with Michelle Obama, the First Lady of the United States of America. I will never forget the beauty that she radiated the night of her husband's inauguration. I appreciate her style, self-confidence, and heart full of love for the military defending our country.

Even so, looking good comes from the inside, not the outside. A heart centered on God makes a woman's face glow as she accomplishes successful living in today's world.

So, if you are 50, rest assured that you are God's, and He has divine ownership of you! He has said, "*Now therefore, if you will obey my voice indeed, and keep my covenant, then ye shall be a peculiar treasure unto me above all people: for all the earth is mine*" (Exodus 19:5 KJV).

• FEELING GOOD •

Start your morning with a prayer like Nehemiah's: "Lord, let Your ear be attentive to the prayer of this Your servant and to the prayer of Your servants who delight in revering Your name. Give your servant success today by granting her favor. (See Nehemiah 1:3.) Thank You for giving me success and favor as I enjoy the gifts of this day. In Jesus' name, amen."

Feeling good begins with great spiritual health, physical health, and mental health. Starting each day with a quiet time spent with your heavenly Father fills you with His power and gives you balance as you go about your day. Welcome the living Word into your heart each morning for successful living. Pray and be consumed with the power of one-on-one communication with the Ruler of the universe. Listen as He speaks to your heart in His still, small voice. He says, "*Be still, and know that I am God; I will be exalted among the nations, I will be exalted in the earth*" (Psalm 46:10 NIV). In today's busy world, it is your responsibility to make a daily habit of connecting personally with the living God.

Along with prayer time, it's important to stay attuned to God's voice throughout the day and to be aware of His beautiful universe that surrounds you. God is "up close and personal." For example, one morning, I was having my quiet time on my patio and watching the sunrise. I was reading God's Word and praising Him when I noticed a baby bluebird perched near me. It warmed my heart and brought tears to my eyes. (My dad, a farmer, dearly loved bluebirds. When I was a child, he would get up early, sit drinking his coffee on the back porch, and watch the bluebirds in the backyard.) My dad is now in heaven; but, that day, I felt his spirit as I watched his favorite bird and enjoyed intimacy with God.

We are made up of body, soul, and spirit. Our "bodysuit" is home for our soul and spirit. Our soul consists of our emotions, will, and intellect. Being a spirit, we have the ability to connect with God's Spirit. Your spirit is the real you! And your real identity is in Christ Jesus. "*God is spirit, and his worshipers must worship in spirit and in truth*" (John 4:24 NIV). You are a spirit-person; therefore, you have the ability to connect with the divine Spirit of God. Your spirit and your soul live in your body. When you see yourself as a child of God and connect your spirit with His Spirit, you have supernatural power. You will radiate holy light through your spirit when it's connected with your Creator.

To keep this miraculous, God-given body exercised and well fed is a huge responsibility of fabulous-after-50 women. If we add to the equation mental fitness, we are now becoming a complete person. With the explosion of knowledge through the Internet, sharpening our mental ability is truly an exciting adventure. We continue to become all that God has created us to be.

As you enjoy your 50th year, do not compare yourself to others, because you are unique. God called each of us to be great in our own way and in our own circle of life. Do you understand the greatness that is within you after 50 years of life? "*This is the day which the LORD hath made; we will rejoice and be glad in it*" (Psalm 118:24 KJV)

Have faith and look up during your maturing years. Remember, "*I can do all things through Him who strengthens me*" (Philippians 4:13).

• DOING GOOD •

Get inspired to make a difference and have the best day ever. You are blessed to bless others.

I was blessed with a lovely, kind, saintly mother who loved me like a princess. During her illness in her later years, I would call her on the phone early in the morning and ask her for a dinner date. She was so excited that she would work all day to look presentable. At 86, she was still wearing stilettos! I would set a certain time to pick her up in my car and drive her to a restaurant of her choice. When I knocked on the door, she would open it and do a little waltz for me, turning so I could see how beautiful she looked. We would enjoy our meal together while keeping the conversation warm with memories, stories of the past, and hope for the future. Now that she is dancing on the streets of gold, I am blessed with memories of her.

With the decline of our economy and the prevalence of natural disaster and wars, the world is fertile with opportunities to be charitable. After 50 is the perfect time in life to reach out and help someone.

Jesus commanded us to *"love one another, as I have loved you"* (John 15:12 KJV). As you live through the decade of your 50s, you'll find no greater joy than helping someone in need—whether that be a friend, a child, or a parent, or a complete stranger. The most gratifying experiences are the heartfelt gifts of love, time, and money given in the name of Jesus. The act of making a significant difference in someone's life or circumstance floods our souls with God's marvelous light. Like the sunshine after a rain, when we look up, we see the beautiful rainbow in the sky. The fifth decade of life is prime time!

• YEAR OF JUBILEE •

In Israel, during every 50th year, the land rested, and the people enjoyed a jubilee.

> *And ye shall hallow the fiftieth year, and proclaim liberty throughout all the land unto all the inhabitants thereof....A jubilee shall that fiftieth year be unto you: ye shall not sow, neither reap that which groweth of itself in it, nor gather the grapes in it of thy vine undressed. For it is the jubilee; it shall be holy unto you.* (Leviticus 25:10, 11–12 KJV)

Likewise, your 50th birthday is a time to embrace triumphs and pivotal points of life changes. Enjoy the second half of life—it's a magnificent celebration!

• QUESTIONS FOR IMMEDIATE APPLICATION •

1. Are you setting some aside time every day to spend with Christ? If not, what could you do to make time?
2. It's important to praise God for the universe that surrounds us every day. What are three things in your world you can praise Him for today?
3. How would viewing the 50th year of life as a Jubilee change the way you approach your relationships and everyday tasks?

• TOP TEN TRUTHS ABOUT BEING 50 •

1. Fifty is the age to live large. Live purposefully, and others will follow.
2. The age of 50 should never be underestimated. Life experience, health, and ambition can make it the zenith of your life!

3. Creating memories with those who are most important to you will bring comfort later on down the road.
4. One of the most gratifying and priceless experiences in life is that of giving of our love, time, and money to others.
5. You do not need to look very far to find an opportunity to be charitable. Take advantage of these opportunities!
6. Making a difference in someone's life will flood your soul with God's marvelous light.
7. Looking good comes from inside—a heart devoted to Christ—not from outside appearances.
8. You have the ability to connect with God's Spirit through His Word. Take advantage of it!
9. When you are connected with the Spirit, you have supernatural power!
10. Don't spend the 50th year of life moping; spend it celebrating the past and looking forward to your glorious future!

AGING SUCCESSFULLY: ATTITUDE #12

As God blesses me with more years, I will invest my experience and energy into the lives of others.

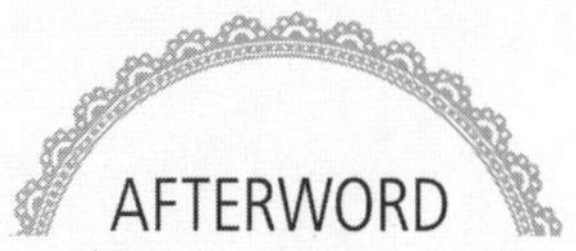

AFTERWORD

T.G.I.F.–THANK GOD I'M 50!

When I reached 50, I felt ripely appreciative. I had survived the tides of disease and accidents. I felt stronger: mentally, physically, socially, and spiritually. I was more self-confident through the power of Jesus Christ and from 50 years of living. I liked being 50-something. I was health conscious, exercising every day.

Noted gerontologist Nathan Shock believes true age changes by a 1 percent decline per year, beginning at age 30. This assumes we are at 100 percent at age 30! My desire is to have at least 90 percent of my total body capacity when I die.

Throughout my 50s, I had unique ideas and a positive attitude. I felt I was at my creative peak! I was not embittered about aging. I planned to grow old in a positive way. I plan to age creatively, energetically, and productively.

Aging is a plus for a writer; age and experience just make me better at my craft. I never feel diminished or declining–I feel as if my career and I are on the launchpad! Now that my wonderful three children are grown and I don't feel confined by the duties of childcare, I am increasing my focus on career. I like this time in my life. The older I get, the more friends I have: spiritual friends, women and men friends, writer friends, and family friends. I feel rich!

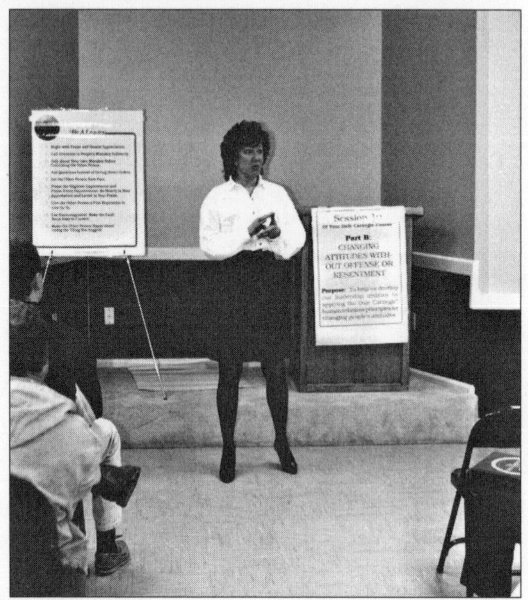

Shirley speaking at a seminar at Dale Carnegie Training

Being older makes me more curious. I crave learning new things. Seeing a new movie, reading a stimulating book, meeting a new person, or listening to different music makes life extraordinary. At last, I have leisure time! Hurray! I like lag time, self-time, and solitude, which is a rare treasure. After raising a wonderful family, I am enjoying this pausal time in life. I am free to *be*. With a solid foundation of family, God, and country, now is the time to build on that foundation.

My desire is to help remove the stigma of aging, so the younger women will not feel depressed as they age.

After finding my rhythm, I do not expect others to be my happiness. I am already happy. I enjoy life; I have my own identity; I like myself. Self-acceptance is priceless.

I am awestruck with the miraculousness of the universe. I am enamored of life. The magnificence of each day is awesome.

The bliss I feel when I look into the angelic faces of my grandchildren fills me with joy. When I witness compassion in action, I am filled with wonder.

I feel a spirit of aliveness within myself. I feel like saying yes to life! Life is an adventure.

With the hope of eternity through my Lord and Savior, Jesus Christ, I am euphoric about the future—mine and yours.

With grace and peace and a spirit of adventure,

Shirley W. Mitchell

ENDNOTES

Chapter 1

1. Dr. Ken Dychtwald, *Age Power* (New York: Jeremy P. Tarcher/ Putnam, 1999), 235.
2. Thomas Arnold, quoted in John P. Bradley, Leo F. Daniels, Thomas C. Jones, and Tryon Edwards, eds., *The International Dictionary of Thoughts* (Chicago, IL: J.C. Ferguson Publishing Co., 1969), 20.
3. Quoted in Frances Weaver, *The Girls with the Grandmother Faces* (New York: Hyperion Books, 1996), 39.
4. Dychtwald, "Age Wave Speaks" 11, no. 4 (November/December 1993): 13.
5. Walter M. Bortz II, M.D., *Dare to Be 100* (New York: Simon & Schuster, 1996), 23.
6. Margaret Sharpe, "More Precious than Gold," *The Shantyman* (January–February 1996): 2.
7. B. F. Skinner, *Enjoy Old Age: A Practical Guide* (New York: W. W. Norton & Co., Inc., 1997), 76–77.

Chapter 2

1. Glenn Van Ekeren, *The Speaker's Sourcebook* (Englewood Cliffs, NJ: Simon & Schuster, 1988), 222.
2. Albert Ellis, Ph.D., and Emmett Velten, Ph.D., *Optimal Aging: Get Over Getting Older* (Chicago/LaSalle, IL: Open Court Publishing Co., 1998), 255.

3. Penne Laubenthal, "Mid-Life Crisis," *The Elk River Review*, 1, no. 2 (December 1992). Used by permission.
4. Weaver, *Girls with the Grandmother Faces*, 43.
5. Quoted in Weaver, *Girls with the Grandmother Faces*, 42.
6. Van Ekeren, *Speaker's Sourcebook*, 64.

Chapter 3

1. Shirley W. Mitchell, *Spiritual Sparks for Busy Women* (Huntsville, AL: Strode Publishers, 1982), 23.
2. Jeannie Williams, "Noonan's Gospel of the Good Life," *USA Today* (10 May 1994): 2D.
3. Paul E. Billheimer, *Destined for the Throne* (Minneapolis, MN: Bethany House Publishers, 1975), 16.

Chapter 4

1. Jane Rubietta, *Quiet Places: A Woman's Guide to Personal Retreat* (Minneapolis, MN: Bethany House Publishers, 1997), 23.
2. J. I. Packer, *Knowing God* (Downers Grove, IL: InterVarsity Press, 1973), 58.
3. "Hallelujah! Long Live the Faithful!" *Health* (October 1999): 30.
4. Billheimer, *Destined for the Throne*, 18.
5. Rubietta, *Quiet Places*, 16.
6. Jane Rubietta, *Still Waters: Finding the Place Where God Restores Your Soul* (Minneapolis, MN: Bethany House Publishers, 1999), 15.

Chapter 5

1. Corrie ten Boom, *In My Father's House* (Carmel, NY: Guideposts, 1976), cover flap.
2. For more on loss, as well as dreams, see Rubietta, *Quiet Places.*
3. Valerie Bell, *She Can Laugh at the Days to Come* (Grand Rapids, MI: Zondervan Publishing House, 1996), 51.
4. From a speech presented at Carmel High School, Libertyville, Illinois, 1999.
5. Joan Rivers, *Don't Count the Candles: Just Keep the Fire Lit!* (New York: HarperCollins, 1999), 146.
6. Thomas Kinkade, *With Wings like Eagles* (Nashville, TN: Thomas Nelson, 1998), 79.
7. Dr. Maxwell Maltz, *Psycho-Cybernetics*, 1996, as quoted in Helen Nearing, ed., *Light on Aging and Dying* (Gardiner, ME: Bilbury House Publishers, 1995), 6.
8. Sam E. Roberts, *Exhaustion: Causes and Treatments* (Emmaus, PA: Rodale Publishing Co., 1967), as quoted in *Reader's Digest* (April 1995): 33.
9. Christiane Northrupp, M.D., *Women's Bodies, Women's Wisdom* (New York: Bantam Books, 1998), 597.
10. Bill Meyers, "Women Increase Standing as Business Owners," *USA Today* (29 June 1999): B1.
11. Rick Boling, "Four Awesome Volunteers," *Modern Maturity* (July–August 1999): 76.
12. Rivers, *Don't Count the Candles*, 152.
13. The Mobile Missionary Assistance Program, composed of Christian Recreational-Vehicle owners, travels and does

projects for various organizations, missionary groups, etc. Contact them at their office in Calimesa, CA, 909-795-3944.

NOMADS (Nomads on a Mission Active in Divine Service) is a newly formed organization within the United Methodist Volunteers in Mission (UMVIM) program, which also travels by RV to mission sites to work. They can be contacted through any local United Methodist Conference office.

14. "Lend a Hand, Live Longer," *Health* (June 1999): 28.

Chapter 6

1. Roy M. Oswald, *Clergy Self-Care: Finding a Balance for Effective Ministry* (Washington, D.C.: The Alban Institute, 1991), 130.
2. Ibid.
3. Abraham Kaplan, *Love…and Death*, 1973, as quoted in Nearing, ed., *Light on Aging and Dying*, 49.
4. Ruth H. Jacobs, *Be an Outrageous Older Woman* (New York: HarperCollins, 1997), 171.
5. Dychtwald, *Age Wave*, 219.
6. Ten Boom, *In My Father's House*, 43.
7. U.S. Bureau of the Census, as quoted in *USA Today* (1 July 1999): 1–2D, 8D.
8. For further work on setting boundaries and caring for your own needs, consult Rubietta, *Quiet Places*.
9. U.S. Bureau of the Census, *USA Today* (1 July 1999).

Chapter 7

1. Walter M. Bortz, M.D., *We Live Too Short and Die Too Long* (New York: Bantam Books, 1991), 201.

2. Tammie Smith, "Age Gracefully," *The Tennessean* (31 August 1999): 5D.
3. According to the Center for the Study of Anorexia and Bulimia in New York City, about 25 percent of patients are over 30; the majority of the people in support groups run by the National Association of Anorexia Nervosa & Associated Disorders, Highland Park, IL, are 30 or older. "Older women with eating disorders fit into three categories: those who have struggled with the disorder since their teens; those who had an early occurrence, but recovered and remained symptom-free until later years; and those whose symptoms first cropped up well past their teen years. Experts also say older women are more likely to be bulimic—to binge and purge, either through vomiting or through the use of laxatives—than they are to be anorexic." Lorna Collier, "The Aging of Anorexia: Middle-aged Women—and Older—Fight the Devastating Disease," *Chicago Tribune* (24 October 1999): 3–4.
4. Bortz, *We Live Too Short and Die Too Long*, 130.
5. Carol Ann Rinzler, "It's Never Too Late for...Foods That Fight Aging," *Reader's Digest* (November 1990): 13.
6. Northrup, *Women's Bodies, Women's Wisdom*, 554.
7. Bortz, *We Live Too Short and Die Too Long*, 130.
8. Patricia Cobe, "The Lowdown on Low Fat," *Your Body, Your Heath* (11 January 1992).
9. Carol A. Chapman, "The Nutrition Evangelist," *Charisma Magazine* (July 1992): 18.
10. Michael Roizen, *RealAge: Are You As Young As You Can Be?* (New York: HarperCollins, 1999), 174.
11. Ibid., 184.

12. Chapman, "The Nutrition Evangelist."

13. Gary Null, *Gary Null's Ultimate Anti-Aging Program* (New York: Kensington Books, 1999), 273.

14. Ibid., 274.

Chapter 8

1. Mike Snider, "U.S. Tends to Take It Easy on Exercise," *USA Today* (2 June 1992).

2. Bortz, *We Live Too Short and Die Too Long*, 191.

3. John W. Rowe, M.D., and Robert L. Kahn, Ph.D., *Successful Aging* (New York: Random House, 1998), 141.

4. Roizen, *RealAge*, 210.

5. Rowe and Kahn, *Successful Aging*, 141.

6. Roizen, *RealAge*, 225.

7. National Institute on Aging, *Exercise*, 33.

8. *Walking Magazine*, 1987.

9. Ibid., 1987, reader profile of 2,900 walkers.

10. Miriam Nelson, Ph.D., "Living to the Max," *Modern Maturity* (July–August 1999): 29–35.

11. National Institute on Aging, *Exercise*, 36.

12. Roizen, *RealAge*, 211.

13. Rowe and Kahn, *Successful Aging*, 47.

14. Roizen, *RealAge*, 238.

15. *Exercise: A Guide from the National Institute on Aging*, Pub. No. NIH 99-4258, 58–70.

16. Ibid., 58.

17. Roizen, *RealAge*, 237–239.

18. Ibid., 213–214.

Chapter 9

1. Gail Sheehy, *New Passages: Mapping Your Life Across Time* (New York: Random House, 1995), 199, 202.
2. *USA Today* (29 October 1993).
3. Robert G. Wells and Mary C. Wells, *Menopause and Midlife* (Wheaton, IL: Tyndale House Publishers, 1994), 26.
4. Gail Sheehy, *The Silent Passage* (New York: Random House Books, 1992), 41.
5. Author's note: stress, illness, and change in weight can also cause temporary cessation of, or change in, menstruation. Don't be misled into thinking you are menopausal (and therefore can't get pregnant!). Check with your specialist to know for sure.
6. Isadore Rosenfeld, M.D., *Live Now, Age Later: Proven Ways to Slow Down the Clock* (New York: Warner Books, Inc., 1999), 190.
7. Author's note: Wells and Wells (*Menopause and Midlife*, 138) state that most bone loss occurs in the first five years after menopause. Sheehy says, "We begin to lose bone after the age of 35; the normal rate of loss is about one percent a year." Epidemiologist Trudy Bush adds, "When you hit 50, bone loss accelerates to about a percent and a half each year for about ten years" (*Silent Passage*, 109). The timing of ERT or HRT is all the more crucial given the silent ramifications of osteoporosis.
8. H. Jick, L. E. Derby, M. W. Myers, et al., *Lancet* 348: 981-883, 1996.
9. Ibid.

10. G. A. Colditz, S. E. Hankinson, et al., *New England Journal of Medicine* (1995): 1589–1593.

11. Author's note: Statistics released by Centers for Disease Control for 1996 rank heart disease as the number one killer, with 733,834 estimated deaths in the United States. Cancer of all types ranked second, with an estimated 544,278 deaths (as cited by Gary Null, Ph.D, in *Gary Null's Ultimate Anti-Aging Program* [New York: Kensington Books, 1999, 125]).

Chapter 10

1. Roald Dahl, *The Twits* (New York: Puffin Books/Viking Penguin, 1991), 9.
2. For more information on Color Me Beautiful locations and consulting options, visit www.colormebeautiful.com/.
3. "10 Anti-Aging Makeup Tricks," *Health* (September 1999): 103.

Chapter 11

1. Bell, *She Can Laugh at the Days to Come*, 57.
2. Bradley, Daniels, Jones, and Edwards, eds., *International Dictionary of Thoughts*, 730.

•●•

CONTRIBUTORS

Jane Rubietta, international speaker and Cofounder of Abounding Ministries, received her Bachelor of Science in Business and attended Trinity Divinity School in Illinois. She is the Assistant Director and Manuscript Coordinator for the Write-to-Publish Conference in Wheaton, Illinois. She is an award-winning author of 11 books, including *Quiet Places, Still Waters* and *Come Along: The Journey into a More Intimate Faith*. For more information, visit www.janerubietta.com.

James Upchurch, M.D., GYN, graduated from the Medical College of Alabama. Following his four years of service in the United States Air Force, in which he assumed the position of Captain, Dr. Upchurch completed an OB-GYN residency and practiced for 32 years in Birmingham. His work has been published in several medical journals, including the American Journal of Obstetrics and Gynecology.

Dr. Debra K. Goodwin, Ph.D., R.D., is an Associate Professor and Department Head of Family & Consumer Sciences at Jacksonville State University in Alabama. She received a B.S. in Administrative Dietetics from Jacksonville State University, an M.A. in Allied Health Education from the University of Alabama, and a Ph.D. in Health Education and Health Promotion from the University of Alabama. Her research interests include adolescent nutrition, women's nutrition, and workplace wellness. She has given numerous presentations and published many articles on adolescent diabetes and menu modification. To contact Dr. Goodwin, email her at dgoodwin@jsu.edu.

•●•

ABOUT THE AUTHOR

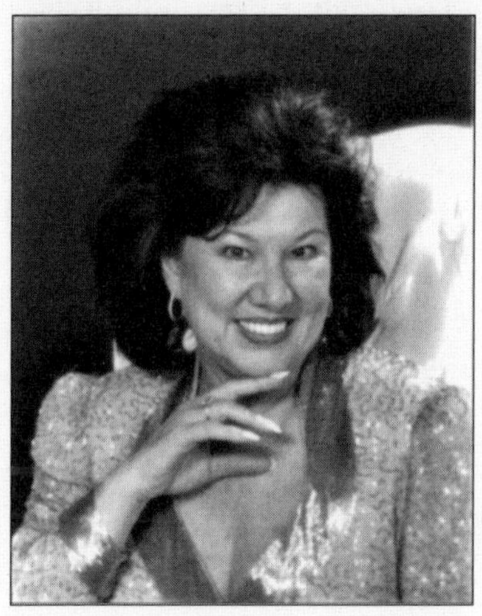

Shirley W. Mitchell
"The Golden Egg of Aging"

Shirley W. Mitchell, Dale Carnegie graduate and member of Toastmasters International, was awarded the 2004 Citizen of the Year Award by the Albertville Chamber of Commerce for her contributions to the betterment of society through local community projects. Her glowing smile won her the most Stunning Smile Award during the 2000 Ms. Senior Alabama pageant, and she won the 1997 Woman of Achievement Award, presented by the Albertville Business and Professional Women's Club. Shirley is basking in the time of her life, following biggest passions: writing, speaking, traveling, and being a mother, grandmother, and great-grandmother.

Shirley attended Dr. Ken Dychtwald's "Age Wave Institute" in New York and Dr. Walter M. Bortz II's seminar "Dare to be 100" in California. She also attends the annual Write-to-Publish Conference at Wheaton College. She has published multiple books, including *The Beauty of Being God's Woman*, *Spiritual Sparks for Busy Women*, and *Fabulous Aging Attitudes*.

Known today as The Golden Egg of Aging, Shirley is the owner of the syndicated media groups Fabulous After 50, Sensational After 60, and Aging Outside the Box. She is the columnist of the syndicated Fabulous After Fifty online column, a featured columnist for *Senior Lifestyle Magazine*, writer of the *Passionate Sparks* online newsletter, and a member of The Lit Chicks Literary Writers Critique Group of Sand Mountain, Alabama.

Shirley is the celebrity radio talk show host of the syndicated radio shows *Aging Outside the Box* and *Christian Spiritual Sparks*.

Her passion is being fabulous at any age.

EXTEND THE IMPACT!

If your group or club is interested in booking Shirley W. Mitchell for an upcoming speaking event, conference, seminar, banquet, workshop, or retreat, please contact the Managing Agent-Producer at:

Lighthouse Coastal Productions
466 Sardis Cutoff Road
Sardis City, AL 35956
agent@lighthousecoastal.com
www.lighthousecoastal.com

www.fabulousafter50.com
www.sensationalafter60.com
www.agingoutsidethebox.net